Wheatgrass Nature's Finest Medicine

Revised Edition

by Steve Meyerowitz

Cleanse ✳ Nourish ✳ Rejuvenate ✳ Heal

Wheatgrass

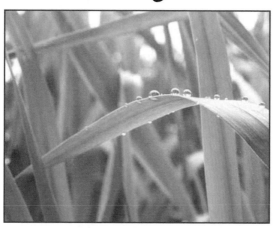

Nature's Finest Medicine

**The Complete Guide to Using Grass
Foods & Juices to Help Your Health**

Revised Edition

by Steve Meyerowitz

Sproutman®

Nutrition ✶ Benefits ✶ Research ✶ History & Religion
Growing ✶ Juicing ✶ Taking ✶ Detoxification ✶ Retreats
Testimonials ✶ Resources ✶ Chlorophyll ✶ Barley Grass

Library of Congress Cataloging-in-Publication Data

Meyerowitz, Steve.
 Wheatgrass : nature's finest medicine : the complete guide to using grass
foods & juices to help your health / by Steve Meyerowitz. –7th ed.
    p. cm.
 Includes bibliographical references and index.
 ISBN-13: 978-1-878736-98-7 (pbk.)
 1. Wheatgrass (Wheat)–Therapeutic use. 2. Vegetable juices–Therapeutic use. 3. Raw foods–Therapeutic use. I. Title.
RM255.M49 2006
613.2'6–dc22
        2006022042

Special thanks to the Int'l Biogenic Society for permission to extract from the
Essene Gospel of Peace by E.B. Szekely. And to the Ann Wigmore
Foundation for permission to use her words in the Epilogue.
Cover photo by Kenneth Crawford, courtesy of Pines International.

Sproutman Publications
PO Box 1100, Great Barrington, Mass. 01230
413-528-5200 Fax 413-528-5201
www.Sproutman.com   Email: info@Sproutman.com

Distributed by
Book Publishing Company
PO Box 99, Summertown, TN 38483
888-260-8458. 931-964-3571 Fax 931-964-3518

Table of Contents

Table of Contents
by Subject

VIII

Dedicated to Charles F. Schnabel

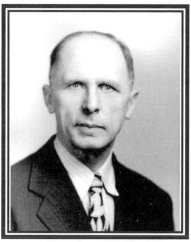

Dr. Charles F. Schnabel
The Father of Wheat Grass
1895–1974

In 1930, Charles F. Schnabel started eating grass. Before anyone else, he initiated a movement to promote the human consumption of grass. He dedicated his entire life to the nutritional and health benefits of grass. He also furthered its role as a premium livestock feed and as a profitable and ecological crop for American farmers. His dream was to see grass included as a valuable supplement to the American diet. He knew from his experiments with animals and his research in the laboratory, that it would boost our nutrition, build good blood, and strengthen our immunity against disease. His vision was of a grass–rich America that would donate tons of grass worldwide to feed the hungry and provide a model for malnourished countries to follow. He is a forgotten hero, but he is remembered in these pages for how close he came to making wheat grass a household food. Few people today are aware of it, but in the 1940s, consumers all over America and Canada could purchase cans of grass in their local pharmacies. Stories about the human consumption of grass appeared in magazines such as Newsweek, Business Week, and Time. Today, grass is only now approaching the level of popularity that Charles Schnabel had crusaded for and achieved over sixty years ago.

This book is dedicated to Dr. Charles F. Schnabel's lifelong and tireless efforts to promote the benefits of grass as a nutritious food. May his dreams come true.

A Wheatgrass Primer

What is Wheatgrass?

Wheatgrass is a variety of grass that is used like an herbal medicine for its therapeutic and nutritional properties. It is available as a fresh squeezed juice, a dried juice concentrate, an extract, a whole leaf powder, or tablets. This book uses the name "wheat" grass because it is the most popular, but the common grains of barley, oat and Kamut grow grasses that are equally potent. *See Spiritual & Religious Roots, History & Culture, Healing with Grass, Nutrition, The Pioneers, Real Stories from Real People.*

What does it do?

It has broad effectiveness, but its three most therapeutic roles are: blood purification, liver detoxification, and colon cleansing. As a food it is very nourishing and restorative with such a complete range of nutrients that it can, by itself, sustain life. This nutritional miracle is most evident in the animal kingdom where studies prove large and small grazing animals not only sustain themselves on young grasses but also improve their health. *See Healing with Grass, Nutrition, Research, Real Stories from Real People, Spiritual & Religious Roots.*

How do I take it?

For therapeutic purposes, you need to take a minimum of six to ten ounces of fresh juice daily or the equivalent in powder. You can also take it rectally through enemas or implants. For nutrition and prevention, you can make powdered drinks or take tablets. *See The Juicers, Healing with Grass, Real Stories from Real People.*

Where do I get it?

From your natural food store, juice bar, direct from growers, or mail order. *See Resources, The Companies, The Pioneers, Wheatgrass Retreats.*

Why should I take it?

Wheatgrass earned its reputation from people with terminal illnesses who took it at the eleventh hour of their lives, after conventional medicine left them with no hope. But you can take it as part of a long range prevention and health maintenance program. *See Healing with Grass, Research, Nutrition, Real Stories from Real People.*

How do I get started?

You can grow the grass yourself, buy it from a grower or health food store, drink the juice at a juice bar or buy bottled grass tablets and powders. But if you are sick, it is highly recommended that you enroll in a wellness program at a wheatgrass retreat center. As an alternative, you can establish a home-health program using the information in this book and the guidance of a knowledgeable health professional. *See Grow Your Own Grass, The Juicers, The Companies, Wheatgrass Retreats.*

Why should I believe you?

There are many scientific studies demonstrating the efficacy and nutrition of grasses. Most information about its therapeutic effectiveness is based on clinical evidence and the word-of-mouth testimony of users. *See Science & Wheatgrass, Research, Real Stories from Real People, Nutrition, Spiritual & Religious Roots, History & Culture.*

Wheat Grass vs. Wheatgrass

A word on spelling. "Wheat grass" is a variety of grass like barley, oats and rye, grown in open fields. "Wheatgrass" refers to the product typically grown indoors in trays and the juice consumed for health maintenance or disease treatment.

Disclaimer

The information in this book is not intended to be a prescription for the user. This book does not offer medical advice and its content has not been evaluated by the US Food and Drug Administration. Instead it presents educational information: research, personal experiences, testimony, and nutritional information regarding the use of plants and vegetables in harmony with natural laws. No information or product described herein should be relied upon implicitly to diagnose, treat, cure, or prevent disease. Please do not read this book if you are unwilling to assume full responsibility for the management of your health. Because each person's condition is unique, the author urges the reader to consult a qualified medical or health professional before undertaking any suggestions described in this book. Good luck and good health.

Acknowledgments

Although my name is placed on the cover of this book, the information presented within comes from a long list of contributors: pioneers, entrepreneurs, researchers, manufacturers, and a few saints. I am grateful to every grower and purveyor mentioned in these pages for their support of my efforts to provide good information to you. What follows is a few special thank you's and the inevitable risk of leaving someone special out.

Thank you to Ron Seibold and the staff of *Pines International*, "the wheat grass people." More than anyone, they carry the torch handed down by Dr. Charles Schnabel of promoting the value of cereal grasses. They do it with quality and integrity. Pines helps return thousands of acres of denatured land to organic soil and donates millions of dollars worth of grass foods to feed the hungry in third world countries. Schnabel would be proud.

Thank you to the *Green Foods Corporation* and the gracious and informative Dr. Bob Terry. Green Foods Corporation has provided a wealth of nutritional and scientific research on barley grass. Founded by Dr. Yoshihide Hagiwara, a living grass foods legend, this company has a strong medical and pharmacological foundation. Hagiwara puts his profits back into research and has added a credibility to grass foods that only science can offer. The entire industry benefits from his work which, in its absence, would depend largely on testimonials.

Thank you to Emily Schnabel-Sloan who took the time and energy to dig through boxes of old papers of her father's work. Thank you to Dick Houston who worked with Dr. Schnabel. Thank you to Julie Irons and her gloriously long memory and to son Robert Irons. Thank you to the *Optimum Health Institute* and the generous and enthusiastic Robert Ross whose photos of wheatgrass grace many of these pages. A thank you to Piter Caizer the "Wheatgrass Messiah," who spreads the message about wheatgrass through his music wherever he goes, and who shines with the powerful energies that grasses and living foods provide. And a thank you to the individuals whose personal experiences with wheatgrass are included in these pages for all to read.

Thank you to Mitchell May of *the Synergy Company* who enthusiastically shared his information and experience to help make this a better book. Thank you to my assiduous proofing editors Nancy Flaxman, Julia

Erickson, Molly Mast, Pauline Clarke and my wife Beth Robbins whose support system was so valuable to me in laboring on this book.

While I cannot thank all the deserving professionals here, I want to take a moment to comment in general on the businesses in the natural products industry. Small manufacturers rarely get their time in the spotlight. Operating in the manic and sometimes ruthless marketplace of the 21st century, consumers can easily develop defensive and even cynical attitudes towards anything commercial. The mere word "corporate," for some, is enough to generate angst. Corporate America has earned this reputation because it raped our lands with dioxin and DDT, polluted our rivers with PCB's, sprayed our vegetables with pesticides and blackened our lungs with cigarettes. Profits before people is its indelible image.

But in direct reaction to this poor record, many younger companies have emerged with purer principles and missions for creating a better world. Often, these companies are formed by visionaries. Integrity matters to them. These are real people with a real desire to make a contribution. They have a dream and their labor is not just about money. I have met many of these entrepreneurs whose dedication to personal and planetary health is exciting. Business is a motivating force in our society—good or bad. It can and has convinced us of the desirability to smoke Marlboro's or eat yoghurt. It is particularly gratifying to see companies promoting back-to-nature concepts and organic whole foods. Not all companies make lots of money—far from it. Small companies spend most of it on research, equipment, processing, packaging, advertising, marketing and employees. When all is said and done, most are not rich. Even the giants in the natural food industry are little fish compared to the whales of mainstream commerce. These hard working natural product companies are helping us improve the quality and the longevity of our lives. To them, I say "thank you."

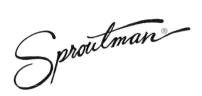

Steve Meyerowitz, Great Barrington, Massachusetts. 2006

History and Culture

The primary form of food is grass. Man's most primeval nutrient, that which nourished him for hundreds of thousands of years, until technological civilization brought with it sprouts, and tender grasses that flourished all over the earth. When man dies, he goes to grass again, and so the tide of life, with everlasting repetition, in continuous circles, moves endlessly on and upward, and in more senses than one, all flesh is grass.

—Edmond Bordeaux Székely [1]

All flesh is grass—Isiah 40/6

We step on it, sit on it, lay on it, jog on it, picnic on it, walk the dog on it, mow it, water it, in fact, we do most everything on it, for it, or with it except eat it! Wherever there is sun, water and earth, there is grass. From the outback down under to the one inch Arctic tundra of Greenland (they call it Greenland) to the hundred foot tropical bamboo, grass is the most fundamental form of vegetation on the planet. Only algae and lichen grow in the extremes of climate that grasses can survive. There are over 9,000 known species of the grass or grain, "gramineae" family. Wheat alone is cultivated on one third of the planet's farm land and grains in general account for half of the world's agriculture.

Grass arrived long before humanity and will undoubtably remain after we have gone. The highest civilizations of the past have coincided with the best grass lands. The Egyptian goddess of fertility Isis, is purported to have discovered the wheat grain in Phoenicia (now Lebanon). The famous Greek historian Herodotus, described this area, the eastern shore of the Mediterranean sea, as the fertile crescent. It is the cradle of Western civilization and a land of unbelievable fertility. Many of our cereal grasses originated here. Ceres (cereal) is what the Romans named the goddess of agriculture. The Greeks used grains as gifts to their goddess of harvest, Demeter and her daughter Persephone. The Chinese honored the cereal grains with elaborate ceremonies conducted as early as 2,800 B.C. The ancient shepherds were nomads and followed the grass season. The prophet and shepherd Isaiah knew how important grass was to humanity: "All flesh is grass and its beauty is like the flowers in the field."[40/6] And the prophet Jeremiah: "Their eyes did fail, because there was no grass."[14/6] Jesus told his followers the humble grass held secrets of heaven and earth and gave birth to all creation. *(See p. 19)* Nebuchadnezzar, King of Babylon, was pitied as a madman when he forsook his palace and ate grass in the meadow. Was he crazy after all? The basic unwritten theme of early human history was the search for greener grass.

What Is Grass?

To a botanist, it is a plant in the gramineae family with narrow leaves, hollow stems and inconspicuous flowers. The leaves are attached to the stems at joints or bulges. Grasses are the most widely distributed group of flowering plants. You'll find them above the Arctic Circle, in temperate and tropical prairies, forests, savannahs, all the way to Antarctica. The "fruit"of grass is grain. Every time you plant a grain, you will grow grass. Wheat, rye, corn, rice, oats, barley, sorghum, millet, spelt, Kamut all make grass. Even the two inch thick sugar cane plant in the tropics and the hundred foot tall bamboo in the Far East are part of the same grass family as the grass on your front lawn. And there are numerous sub-species. Wheat, for example, is part of the genus "triticum," along with oats, barley and rye. It has varieties such as hard wheat, soft, winter, spring, red, gold, durum, semolina, and so forth. Wheat and its sister grains throw out shoots and roots so tightly that they are matted like a green carpet and thus ideal for lawns. When growing it at home in a tray, you can lift the grass out just like a rug. In fact, these root systems can represent up to 90% of the plant's weight[2] enabling grasses to endure drought, cold and even fire. Compare their resilience after a frost to the vegetables in your garden. Can this fortitude be an indicator of its nutritional powers?

Its ubiquity is commensurate with its eminence.

The Cultural Significance of Grass

Grasses are of vast ecological and economic importance. They have been a dominant source of human food throughout history. Grains are a concentrated source of carbohydrates, B vitamins, fatty acids, minerals, fiber and protein. They have migrated with our species from ancient times and places to the modern world. In fact, one quarter of the grass species in the northeastern United States today arrived with European settlers.[3] All the world's cereal crops are grasses and four of the world's top five crops are cereals: wheat, corn, rice and barley. The family also provides most of the world's sugar from sugarcane. Grasses are the primary source of food for domestic and wild grazing animals, which feed on pastures and grasslands. Of the fifteen major crops that feed animals the earth over, ten are grasses. One third of the planet is covered by grass and even in the cemented cities across America, grass fights back through the sidewalk cracks. Its ubiquity is commensurate with its eminence. Nevertheless, we largely ignore it. We chase after the azaleas, roses and orchids instead.

Modern History

Prior to the late 1800's, grass was just known for being a good live-stock feed. But farmers have long observed a qualitative difference in the pelts of livestock that pastured on the young grasses of the early spring. Botanists studied grasses to determine which varieties would produce the healthiest cattle with the highest quality milk, butter and cheese. Animals don't know anything about vitamins. They determine the nutritive value with their instinct, palate and olfactory faculties acting for them in place of judgement. "The preferences shown by cattle are better proofs than those obtained from the analysis of the chemist," said George Sinclair in 1869.[4]

The first documented study of young grass was in 1883 when researchers found that "immature" grass was high in protein and low in fiber.[5] In an analysis that hinted at the jointing theory to be written decades later, an 1890 state agricultural report announced that the mineral matter of grass reached a peak during the period of most rapid growth and declined with maturity.[6] After that, there were no more additions to our knowledge of young grasses on record for forty years. During this time research focused on legumes as the possible answer to our nutritional needs. "Corn is king and alfalfa is queen" was a familiar slogan of the time.

In 1925, an English botanist determined that "young pasture plants are equivalent to protein concentrates." Unfortunately this work lumped together all field grasses, young legumes and young grasses and no distinction was made.[7]

In 1931, Charles F. Schnabel made two discoveries that would change our conceptions about the place of grass in agriculture and initiate the trend for its human consumption. *(See Pioneers, p. 23)* 1: Schnabel demonstrated that a culm of grass reached its peak nutritional value on the day the first joint begins to form. This marks the end of the vegetative stage and the beginning of the reproductive stage of the plant. 2: The food value of the grass at the jointing stage roughly paralleled its protein content. He found that grass grown on richly fertilized land would produce 40% protein grass. This represented a miraculous food value in terms of the agricultural resources and economics necessary to produce protein through other animal and vegetable sources.

In the 1940's, Schnabel inspired the large scale production of young cereal grasses that were dehydrated, canned and sold as nutritional supplements in pharmacies throughout North America. In fact, cereal grass tablets were the nations best selling multiple vitamin and mineral supplements. It wasn't until the early 1950's that it was dethroned by the popular *One-A-day Multiple* vitamins and *Geritol.* These products capitalized on the movement towards technology. "Better Living Through Chemistry" was a common slogan of the time, and "man-made" superceded "nature–made" in importance. Science can make bigger fruit with plant hormones, more profits per acre thanks to fertilizers and rid the land of pests with pesticides. These techniques did indeed increase food production, but at the expense of our health and the purity of our soil, water and air.

In the 1970's Dr Ann Wigmore opened Hippocrates Health Institute in Boston, nourishing terminally ill patients back to health with fresh squeezed wheatgrass juice. Today, virtually every natural food store in North America carries a grass foods product whether it be fresh or dried, wheat or barley or Kamut.

Of the numerous tribes of vegetables which clothe and embellish the earth, none is more interesting nor more extensively useful than the natural order gramineae or family of grasses...the food of man, as well as that of the more useful animals, entirely depends on the produce of our corn fields and pastures.
—George Sinclair, 1869[8]

Spiritual & Religious Grass Roots

Wheatgrass in the Dead Sea Scrolls, Ancient Hebrew & Chinese, Modern Messiah's Spiritual Message

*I believe a leaf of grass is no
less than the journey-work of the stars.*
—Walt Whitman[1]

When I touch grass, I touch infinity. It existed long before there were human beings on the earth, and it will continue to exist for millions of years to come. Through the grass, I talk to the Infinite, which is only a silent force. This is not a physical contact. It is not in the earthquake, wind, or fire. It is the invisible world of nature of which I, too, am a part. —George Washington Carver[2]

Grass, we have seen, has had a long and essential relationship with humans and animals among various cultures throughout history and across the globe. But as we explore deeper into ancient times, cultural and historical records gradually merge with religious history and even mysticism. This chapter establishes a foundation for the relevance and importance of grass in modern times by exploring its religious, mystical and spiritual roots. Specifically, we will look at the definition of grass in the characters of the ancient Hebrew and Chinese languages, listen to Jesus discuss grass with his disciples and hear a modern day "messiah's" view on the spiritual powers of grass.

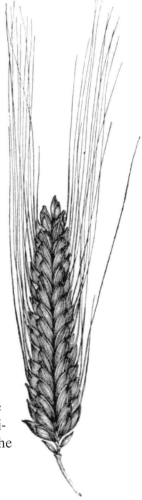

Duham Wheat

The Meaning of "Grass" in Ancient Hebrew and Chinese

Language is very telling. Etymologists spend entire careers tracing a language's original meaning and form. At first blush, it is tempting to assume their work belongs to the domain of museums and Universities, but there are often incredible treasures locked inside language that reveal ancient wisdom and enlighten us, even in today's age of progress and technology.

Ancient Chinese was derived from wall pictures, or hieroglyphs, either painted or carved. Some epigraphs on shells go back 3,500 years. But the first cataloging of Chinese symbols into a language began about 2,800 years ago. A single distinctive symbol represents each word in the language and it takes a vocabulary of about 10,000 characters to read a newspaper. The word for grass in Chinese is a picture of two people kneeling at an alter and praying with heads and arms raised skyward.[3]

Ancient Hebrew, the language in which most of the old testament of the Bible was written, has records from the epoch of King David and Solomon, some 3,200 years ago. Prior to that, the language had roots in Phoenician and Canaanite scripts and hieroglyphs.

In Joe Sampson's book, *Written By the Finger of God—Decoding Ancient Languages*[4], he describes Hebrew as the word of God handed down with a sacred message in each and every character. The Hebrew characters, he says, contain an incredible amount of compressed and layered meaning—a literal spiritual code distilled in every character. The oldest form of the Hebrew word grass is *"Deshe"* spelled דאשכ ך *Dalet,* ש *Shin,* א *Aleph.* One interpretation of this Hebrew code would be:

Through the lowest of the kingdoms on earth is the doorway through which we may be regenerated and come towards perfection of being.[5]

What is the message encoded in the Hebrew word for grass thousands of years ago? Is it regeneration? A path toward perfection? Is grass the primary herb (Esev) for healing humanity? Modern researchers have defined it as a complete food. Can people live on grass? Why does the life–giving nourishment trapped inside its blades provide health and longevity to guinea pigs, rabbits and hens *(see Pioneers)*, while a diet of alfalfa, lettuces and other greens leaves them emaciated and sick?[6] How can 2,000 pound grazing animals, cattle, deer, horses, bison, buffalo, antelopes, elephants, gazelles and giraffes all live and thrive on an exclusive diet of grass? Will grass provide the nourishment people need as well? Can what the chemists call the "unidentified factors" or "grass-juice factors" promote our recovery from sickness and disease? Can the blood rejuvenating chlorophyll held within its leaves restore our natural health and longevity?

The Spiritual Powers of Grass
A Conversation with Piter U. Caizer, The Wheatgrass Messiah

Piter U. Caizer is a German born musician who was disheartened by the excessive use of drugs and alcohol in the rock music world. Major music celebrities who influence millions were too important to destroy themselves and present the wrong example to others. So Piter decided to do something about it. He brought his juicer wherever he would play and made green juices for everyone. "After playing for hours, musicians get dizzy and tired. So instead of doing drugs and going down, they're doing live foods and going up." He turned everyone "on" and they experienced the long-term energy boost of live green juice. The musicians called him "the Wheatgrass Messiah." His special perspective of why wheatgrass works follows here in his own words.[7]

Philosophy of Living Foods

If you think about assimilation of sunlight, humans don't take the energy directly from the sun; we're going through other sources—green plants. We should develop a diet that gets closer to the foods that provide that energy, but instead we have gone in the opposite direction with highly cooked, fried, microwaved, processed food and it's all dead. It doesn't provide any vitality. For me it's about vitality. Food has to give me vitality. When I eat food I want to feel energetic and happy and good. When I eat cooked food, I feel tired. It just doesn't work. You eat dead food and it brings your vibration down and your body has to wrestle with it, to get it out of the system, then you come back up. Then you eat again and it goes down again. So if you eat live food, your vibration doesn't go down; it gets higher and higher and you grow in a spiritual way.

> *Wheatgrass contains raw chlorophyll. Chlorophyll is condensed sunlight. Since we are light beings, spirit and soul inside solid bodies, the light force vibrates through the physical body. That's the energy you feel. That's why wheatgrass is a spiritual food. It nourishes you on the spiritual level as well as the physical.*

Rocket Fuel

When I learned about the grasses and what they can do for you, I said "this is it." Now we have got to find a way to make it palatable because if you give people tray-grown wheatgrass, they say "...uhh, I don't like this." So I worked on the taste. The first thing I mix in my wheatgrass juice is sunflower sprouts. Because sunflower, if you look at the plant, is an amazing plant. It is almost standing human-like with its radiating big face. Sunflower seed is a complete protein. The wheatgrass doesn't have a lot of protein, so by mixing the two together I make it more complete and wow, what an improvement in the taste! So much better, you get a little nutty taste in there from the sunflower sprouts. Then I add some lettuce, and parsley, ginger, beets, celery and alfalfa sprouts. Put in whatever you want. All of a sudden you have this mixture which tastes great and has the benefits of all the individual ingredients mixed together in this dynamic energy juice—I call it rocket fuel.

If you think about the human body like a car, then I want to give it the best fuel I can get. If you go to the gas station you can choose between premium, regular and low octane. Jet fuel is the highest octane. Well, wheatgrass is like jet fuel for humans. It's the best fuel you can get. And, because it goes right into your system, you can feel it. I give green juice to a depressed person and their depression goes away. How is that possible? Because they get back into that harmonious field that we all have deep inside, and you feel in balance; you feel in touch with Mother Nature again. But if you eat all these fried foods, microwaved, you're going the opposite way. You're going out of touch with our nature and we cannot survive apart from nature. We are a part of Mother Nature.

Spiritual Growth

We are vibrating beings with invisible spirit–soul bodies inside us. So when you drink grass juice, what happens? It elevates your vibration and you become more aware that there is something higher going on that is not perceptible with the physical senses but which can be perceived with the higher senses which are dormant within us. We have to make an effort to wake up through meditation and concentration; to activate these spiritual senses which are deep within us. But the way our society runs, everything is all 'outside, outside,' and people spend their time running around wasting their lifetimes making money instead of developing consciousness. When we die the only thing we take with us is our consciousness from when we were in the flesh. The more you can develop that, the more you can actively work on your evolution.

Anti-Aging

We talked about chlorophyll. Chlorophyll is as close to the molecular structure of human blood as anything on the planet. So you can actively revitalize your blood. From an external source comes a raw material that the body can instantly convert into fresh blood. We're only as healthy as our blood is. So, the more you can rejuvenate the blood, the more you slow down the aging clock.

First they cook it, then they freeze it, then they microwave it. What is left in it? That's dead. I wouldn't even give it to my dog.

The older you grow, the more you burn up your natural enzymes and the harder it is to digest your food. That creates all kinds of complications in the body. People have all this accumulated, incompletely digested stuff in there because they can't secrete enough enzymes anymore. The linings of the intestines are all plugged up. If you look at the average diet of what people eat, it's loaded with heavy foods like cheeses and meats...sure you can get away with it for some years but look at the big picture, look at all the people hidden away in the hospitals. And what do they do with them? Instead of relieving their toxicity and cleaning them out, they feed them drugs, making them even more toxic. That whole approach just doesn't work.

Then you have people in their fifties that look young. They have this beautiful energy radiating from them because they are doing that transformation within them. Then you look at others and they look hard and stiff. The difference between youth and age is in the flexibility. Age brings solidity. So when you do the juices and the wheatgrass, you don't experience that because you are constantly replenishing your system with the energy of youth from the young grass. So your system is not growing old as much because it is not burning out as much. It's like a bank account. If you constantly draw money out of it, you are eventually going to go bankrupt. That is exactly what the others are doing to their bodies, they are bankrupting their health. They're eating corrosive food, then their bodies become corroded, then their minds become corroded. They're getting old because they are rusting!

We've got to empty the hospitals. In the Chinese way, the doctor is paid to keep you healthy. Once you get sick, he doesn't get paid because he didn't do his job right. That is what is wrong with our medical profession. They don't teach the people to help themselves and heal. In the whole medical profession there is one word they don't use; it's *heal*.

We are all one. We are all from the same ocean. We are all drops of that same ocean. And we only can come back together in the spirit, in the consciousness; we cannot come back together in our opinions because everyone has opinions but we can come together in the truth. And the truth will always be the truth, it cannot be altered by man. And that is what is so beautiful about the truth. No one can change the truth. The truth will always be the truth. And what is the truth about sprouts and wheatgrass will always be the truth, now and in a thousand years.[8]

The superior physician helps before the early budding of disease...To administer medicines to diseases which have already developed is comparable to the behavior of those persons who begin to dig a well after they have become thirsty.
—Huang Ti, 2697–2597 B.C. legendary Chinese ruler and cultural hero known as "The Yellow Emperor" who co-founded Taoism with Lao-Tsu.

Jesus' Words from the Essene Gospels

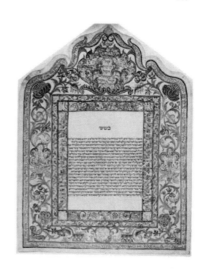

The most precious gift of your Earthly Mother is the grass beneath your feet...
—Jesus, the Essene Gospel of Peace IV[9]

The Essene Gospels represent an exciting piece of history and a timeless message of healing, peace and love. The Essenes were a Jewish sect who lived with Jesus near the Dead Sea. They preserved his words on leather scrolls which were left behind in caves and found generations later after they had fled from Palestine. Some of these scrolls were excavated between 1946 and 1951 and are called the *Dead Sea Scrolls.* The Gospels are translated directly from the Aramaic dialect spoken by Jesus. Thus the translation has a purity and simplicity that remains powerful even in modern times. The following, extracted from the *Discovery of the Essene Gospel of Peace*, by Dr. Edmond Bordeaux Székely, describes in part, the story of how the scrolls were left in the Dead Sea:

"They sent out healers. And one of them was Jesus, the Essene. He walked among the sick and the troubled, and he brought them the knowledge they needed to cure themselves. Some who followed him wrote down what passed between him and those who suffered and were heavy-laden. The Elders of the Brotherhood made poetry of the words, and made unforgettable the story of the Healer of Men, the Good Shepherd. And when the time came at last for the Brothers to leave the desert and go to another place, the scrolls stayed behind as buried sentinels, as forgotten guardians of eternal and living truth.

"A dark age began, a time of savagery, of barbarism, of book-burning, of superstition and worship of empty idols. The gentle Jesus was lost forever in the image of a crucified God; the Essene brothers hid their teachings in the minds of the few who could preserve them for their descendants, and the Scrolls of Healing lay neglected beneath the shifting shadows of the desert..."

About Edmond Bordeaux Székely

Edmond Bordeaux Székely is a well known translator and philologist (scholar of languages). He was a professor of Sanskrit, Aramaic, Greek and Latin, and spoke ten modern languages. His grandfather, Alexandre Székely, was the eminent poet and Unitarian Bishop of Cluj. He is also a descendant of Csoma de Körös, the Transylvanian who compiled the first English-Tibetan dictionary. In addition to translating selected texts from the Dead Sea Scrolls, Edmond B. Székely spent half of the 1920's secluded in the Secret Archives of the Vatican. There, as the result of limitless patience, faultless scholarship and unerring intuition, he discovered and translated the Aramaic scrolls known today as the Essene Gospels.

The first book of the *Essene Gospel of Peace*, published in 1934, has sold over five million copies with no commercial advertisement, and has been translated into twenty-six languages. Book Two, *The Unknown Books of the Essenes* and Book Three *The Lost Scrolls of the Essene Brotherhood* were published almost fifty years later. Book Four, *The Teachings of the Elect*, from which the following is extracted, was published posthumously in 1981 according to Dr. Székely's wishes. They represent yet another fragment of the complete manuscript which exists in Aramaic in the Secret Archives of the Vatican and in Old Slavonic in the Royal Library of the Hapsburgs in Austria. The poetic style of the translations brings to vivid reality the exquisitely beautiful words of Jesus and the Elders of the Essene Brotherhood. The chapter quoted from here is called *"The Gift of the Humble Grass."* Some of the other chapters are: *The Essene Communions, The Sevenfold Peace, The Holy Streams of Life, Light, and Sound. The International Biogenic Society,*[10] founded in 1928 by Dr. Székely with Nobel Prize-winning author Romain Rolland, survives today.

Székely was so taken with the reverence Jesus and others devoted to grass, he encouraged its use throughout his teachings. During his life, his workshops were always adorned by the presence of grass pots to "charge" the environment for learning. He called them "biogenic batteries." Students would hold them to absorb their healing, restorative, and life-giving properties. The following extracted text reveals some of the reasons why.

Extract: the Essene Gospel of Peace Book IV

by Edmond Bordeaux Székely

Speaking about the angel of air, water and sun to his Brothers of the Elect round about him, Jesus spoke:

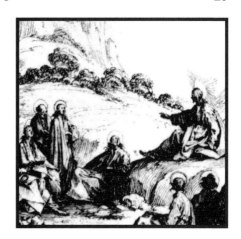

"But of all these, and more, that most precious gift of your Earthly Mother is the grass beneath your feet, even that grass which you tread upon without thought. Humble and meek is the angel of Earth, for she has no wings to fly, nor golden rays of light to pierce the mist. But great is her strength and vast is her domain, for she covers the earth with her power, and without her the Sons of Men would be no more, for no man can live without the grass, the trees and the plants of the Earthy Mother. And these are the gifts of the angel of Earth to the Sons of Men.

"Here is the secret, Sons of Light; here in the humble grass. Here is the meeting place of the Earthly Mother and the Heavenly Father; here is the Stream of Life which gave birth to all creation.

"Behold, Sons of Light, the lowly grass. See wherein are contained all the angels of the Earthly Mother and the Heavenly Father. ...For in the grass are all the angels. Here is the angel of Sun, here in the brightness of the green color of the blades of wheat. For no one can look upon the sun when it is high in the heavens, for the eyes of the Son of Man are blinded by its radiant light. And it is for this that the angel of Sun turns to green all that to which she gives life, that the Son of Man may look upon the many and various shades of green and find strength and comfort therein. I tell you truly, all that is green and with life has the power of the Angel of Sun within it, even these tender blades of young wheat.

"And so does the angel of Water bless the grass, for I tell you truly, there is more of the angel of Water within the grass than any of the other angels of the Earthly Mother...."

"Know also, that the angel of Air is within the grass, for all that is living and green is the home of the angel of Air. Put your face close to the grass, breathe deeply, and let the angel of Air enter deep within your body. For she abides in the grass, as the oak abides in the acorn, and as the fish abides in the sea.

"It is the angel of Life that flows through the blades of grass into the body of the Son of light, shaking him with her power. For the grass is Life and the Son of Light is Life, and Life flows between the Son of Light and the blades of grass, making a bridge to the Holy Stream of Light which gave birth to all creation....

"The Earthly Mother is she who provides for our bodies, for we are born of her, and have our life in her. So does she provide for us food in the very blades of grass we touch with our hands. For I tell you truly, it is not only as bread that wheat may nourish us. We may eat also of the tender blades of grass. That the strength of the Earthy Mother may enter into us. But chew well the blades, for the Son of Man has teeth unlike those of the beasts, and only when we chew well the blades of grass can the angel of Water enter our blood and give us strength. Eat, then, Sons of Light, of this most perfect herb from the table of our Earthly Mother, that your days may be long upon the earth, for such finds favor in the eyes of God.

"I tell you truly, the angel of Power enters into you when you touch the Stream of Life through the blades of grass. For the angel of Power is as a shining light that surrounds every living thing just as the full moon is encircled by rings of radiance and as the mist rises up from the fields when the sun climbs in the sky....

"Touch, then, the blades of grass and feel the angel of Power enter the tips of your fingers, flow upwards through your body, and shake you till you tremble with wonder and awe.

"Know, also, that the angel of Love is present in the blades of grass, for love is in the giving, and great is the love given to the Sons of Light by the tender blades of grass. For I tell you truly, the Stream of Life runs through every living thing, and all that lives, bathes in the Holy Stream of Life. And when the Son of Light touches with love the blades of grass, so do the blades of grass return his love, and lead him to the Stream of Life where he may find life everlasting....

"Touch the blades of grass, Sons of Light, and touch the angel of Eternal life. For if you look with the eyes of the spirit, you will truly see that the grass is eternal. Now it is young and tender, with the brightness of the newborn babe. Soon it will be tall and gracious, as the sapling tree with its first fruits. Then it will yellow with age, and bow its head in patience, as lies the field after the harvest. Finally, it will wither,...but it does not die, for the brown leaves return to the angel of Earth, and she holds the plant in her arms and bids it sleep, and all the angels work within the faded leaves and lo, they are changed and do not die but rise again in another guise. And so do the Sons of Light never see death, but find themselves changed and risen to everlasting Life.

"And so does the angel of Work never sleep, but sends the roots of the wheat deep into the angel of Earth, that the shoots of tender green may overcome death and the reign of Satan. For life is movement and the angel of work is never still....Touch the blades of grass, and thereby touch the Stream of Life. Therein you will find Peace, the Peace built with the power of all the angels. Even so with that Peace will the rays of Holy Light cast out all darkness.

"When the Sons of Light are one with the Stream of Life, then will the power of the blades of grass guide them to the everlasting kingdom of the Heavenly Father. And you shall know more of those mysteries which is not yet time for you to hear. For there are other Holy Streams in the everlasting kingdoms; I tell you truly, the heavenly kingdoms are crossed and crossed again by streams of golden light, arching far beyond the dome of the sky and having no end. And the Sons of Light shall travel by these streams for ever, knowing not death, guided by the eternal love of the Heavenly Father. And I tell you truly, all these mysteries are contained in the humble grass, when you touch it with tenderness and open your heart to the angel of Life within.

"...For so were your fathers taught of old, even our Father Enoch. Go now, and peace be with you."[11]

Grass is the Forgiveness of Nature

Poem by John J. Ingalls, 1898 [12]

Grass is the forgiveness of nature. Lying in the sunshine among the buttercups, daisies and dandelions of May, our earliest recollections are of grass. Grass is the forgiveness of nature, her constant benediction.

....Its tenacious fibers hold the earth in its place and prevent its soluble components from washing into the wasting sea. It invades the solitude of deserts, climbs the inaccessible slopes and the forbidding pinnacles of mountains, modifies climates, and determines the history, character, and destiny of nations. Unobtrusive and patient, it has immortal vigor and aggressiveness.

Banished from the thoroughfares and the fields, it abides its time to return, and when vigilance is relaxed or the dynasty has perished, it silently resumes the throne from which it has been expelled, but which it never abdicated. It bears no blazonry of blooms to charm the senses with fragrance or splendor, but its homely hue is more enchanting than the lily or the rose. It yields no fruit in earth or air and yet, should its harvest fail for a single year, famine would depopulate the world.

Jeremiah 14/6:   "Their eyes did fail, because there was no grass."

Isaiah 40/6:   "All flesh is grass and its beauty is like the flowers
                  in the field."

The Pioneers

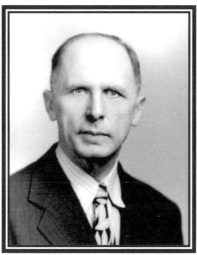

Charles Franklin Schnabel
The Father of Wheat Grass

15 lbs. of wheat grass is equal in overall nutritional value to 350 pounds of ordinary garden vegetables. We have not even scratched the surface of what grass can mean to man in the future.[1] —Charles F. Schnabel

July 31, 1930 was an important day in the history of grass foods. On that day, Charles F. Schnabel got 126 eggs from 106 hens. Anyone who knows about chickens will tell you that those are phenomenal results. To make it even more of a tall story, the hens were sick and dying when Schnabel got them. He only took them to save them from extermination. What does this have to do with grass? To restore their health, Schnabel fed them a mixture of fresh cut, young oat grasses and greens. His miraculous results inspired him to test it on himself. He dried the young greens on his wood stove, powdered them and added them to his family's meals. He had a large family and everyone, including relatives and neighbors, were fed Schnabel's grass. To this day, his daughter still remembers the smell of drying grass that filled the entire house. Such was the beginning of the human consumption of grass in modern times. From this point forward, man has continuously consumed young grasses. Commercial enterprises, thanks to Schnabel, have produced and packaged young grasses. This was the beginning and this was the man who started it.

Schnabel was an agricultural chemist. He specialized in soil fertility, animal feeds and protein research. In the 1920's he worked for the Standard Milling Company and the Kansas Department of Agriculture. So when the depression came and he was laid off in 1930, he had the time and the skills to nurse dying hens back to health. The next spring, he repeated his tests with the hens. Again, the results were striking. Egg production doubled. The eggs had stronger shells and the newborn chicks were free of the common diseases. Even a child could see the difference in their feathers. The grass eating hens averaged 89% productivity while the alfalfa hens averaged 40% productivity. These hens received the same mash and grain ration as the others but with alfalfa added instead of grass.

No one ever heard of such consistently high productivity. Not only that, the mortality rate of the alfalfa hens was ten times greater than the grass hens. In the laboratory he found out why: "The most striking thing was the appearance of their livers which were a dark mahogany color and the surface glistened like a mirror. The alfalfa fed hens had light tan colored livers. These liver changes caused by good grass are too obvious not to have some connection with the prevention of degenerative disease."[2]

Schnabel knew that there was something really potent in the young grass and he immediately started promoting his discovery to feed mills, chemists and the food industry. In the years that followed, he saw his experiments confirmed in the laboratory with chickens, turkeys, rats, rabbits and guinea pigs. Research chemists from major universities identified all known vitamins in grass (except vitamin D) including the newly discovered vitamin K and unnamed nutrients known as the "grass juice factors." *(See Nutrition chapter)* His discovery of the "jointing stage" or the ideal time to harvest grass for maximum nutrition was approved for patents by the USA Patent Office. Large corporations such as Quaker Oats and American Dairies Incorporated invested millions of dollars in further

---

BUSINESS WEEK
June 8, 1940

GRASS, BUT NOT HAY

Butchers, bakers, growers and processors of nearly every description of foodstuff have been finding green pastures under the spreading vitamin tree. And, as everybody must know by now, the green pastures are no longer figurative, since grass itself has shot up to the dignity of a health food.

Cerograss and Cerophyl—the trade names for dehydrated cereal grasses—have received such reams of unsolicited publicity that, novelty or no novelty, business is taking notice.

research and the production of products for animals and humans. Rockhurst College bestowed on him an honorary Doctorate of Science for services to humanity. Bakers made grass enriched breads; the AMA approved grass as a "food," and by 1940, just ten years after his sick hens recovered, cans of Dr. Schnabel's grass were for sale in major drug stores all across the United States and Canada.

Ultimately however, the commercial success of his grass would be short lived. Cerophyl Laboratories of Kansas City, Missouri was the company formed by Quaker Oats and American Dairies for the sale of young cereal grass for human consumption as a drug store nutritional supplement and as a livestock and poultry feed. The name was an abbreviation for chlorophyll from cereal grains. The Green Melk Company, Ltd. was their Canadian counterpart headquartered in Guelph, Ontario. More than 100 persons were employed in Kansas City. But the end of WWII created a widespread materialistic euphoria that diluted public emphasis on personal nutrition. Quaker Oats dropped out, and by 1945 Schnabel was seeking new associations. Unfortunately, the financial and marketing clout of large corporations is required to maintain a product in the national arena and Schnabel never replicated that commercial success.

Despite the successful mass distribution of grass, Schnabel didn't make much money. He was not in it for the money. His goal was to eliminate hunger and malnutrition and he believed grass could do it. His plan proposed a 4 part system: 1. The soil must be reclaimed and enriched. 2. A network of nutritional grass farmers would grow 40% protein grass at greater profit than other crops. 3. A new industry would emerge to properly process, dehydrate, bottle and distribute the grass. 4. Consumers would benefit from a low cost naturally balanced concentrated source of vitamins. Schnabel made extensive calculations as to how many farmers it would take, how many acres, the cost per delivery

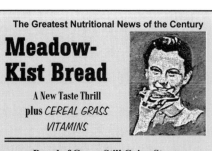

The Greatest Nutritional News of the Century

Meadow-Kist Bread

A New Taste Thrill
plus *CEREAL GRASS VITAMINS*

Bread of Grass. Still Going Strong

Zinsmaster Baking Co. put the emerald-colored loaf on the market in October and reported that first-week sales were the best ever recorded by the firm for any new product. This bread contains virtually every known vitamin except D with a whole alphabet of those undiscovered in its grass-juice factor. The bread was first offered in Duluth where it went like wildfire. The powder also called Meadow-Kist, is made by Doughboy Mills, Inc. and is packaged as a drug-store item, too. —**Business Week 2/1/1941**

THE KANSAS CITY STAR

KANSAS CITY, APRIL 8, 1940—MONDAY

GRAZE YOUR WAY TO HEALTH
CHEMISTS AND STAFF THRIVE ON POWDERED GRASS
New Food Has More Vitamins than the Alphabet has Letters

Fortified physically as well as professionally with grass, three Kansas City chemists left today for Cincinnati to tell the American Chemical society's convention that grass is man's best food. Grass is so full of vitamins the alphabet hasn't enough letters to name them all. Four years of experimenting in the Cerophyl laboratories convinced Charles Schnabel, Dick Graham and George Kohler of that.

Meanwhile, for many months, the three chemists have eaten grass and for several weeks the entire laboratory staff of eighteen persons has had grass luncheons. The powdered grass is put in stews, biscuits, muffins, macaroni, noodles and even candy bars. A 3 year test tube attack revealed grass contains almost all vitamins except D which normally is suppled to grass eating animals by

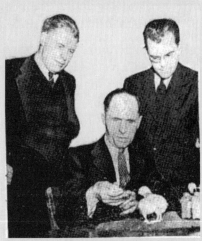

Chemists say Grass is Man's Best Food (l–r) Dr. WR Graham, CF Schnabel and GO Kohler.

sunlight. A parade of vitamins showed up in the grass. Then there was the "grass juice factor" accounting for some food values the vitamins hadn't included. Vitamin K from the grass products was recently found to have blood congealing powers and is being used medically. The paper to be read Wednesday to the chemical convention by Dr. Kohler will claim grass contains vitamins in far richer amounts than fruits and vegetables. A Kansas City obstetrician who used the powders in treating cases of female illness has reported favorably on the effects. At the Mayo clinic, groups of interns have used the powder in experiments. Grass powder as fortification for human diet is definitely proved, Dr. Graham believes and may mean a new cheap way to afford better nutrition.

of those nutrients with grass as compared to other foods. He maintained that high protein (40%) grass was the most profitable crop a farmer could grow based on its market value as a fertilizer, an animal feed and a human nutritional supplement.

What is Schnabel's legacy? While he had much success, he also had many struggles. It was hard to preach about such lofty ideas as ending famine and hidden hunger to a post-war, post-depression era public that was bent on consumerism. Schnabel made several presentations before the American Chemical Society, but he was not a writer. There are no books by him and the few papers and pamphlets he wrote were published mostly in small agricultural and nutritional magazines or regional news-papers. He achieved virtually no fame, his name being lost behind the corporations that produced his ideas or the scientists that published the research on them. But the legacy of his life is fourfold.

First, he inspired a body of scientific research on grass that remained unprecedented until the 1980s. In this, Schnabel was greatly assisted by his colleague, George Kohler. Kohler was a biochemist at the College of Agriculture, University of Wisconsin, Madison. Together with Conrad A. Elvehjem and E.B. Hart, they were the most active group substantiating the food value of cereal grasses in the 1930s and 1940s. This was a prestigious lab. It produced the discovery of Niacin (vitamin B3) by Elvehjem in 1936 which prevents the deficiency disease pellagra. Most significant in their research was the discovery of the "grass juice factor" which indicated that the health improvement powers of grass were distinct from any known vitamins. Kohler was so impressed by the potency of young grass that he moved to Kansas City and worked with Schnabel for several years.

Secondly, Schnabel discovered and patented the jointing theory. To just eat grass was not enough. The secrets of grass's nutritional and healing powers have much to do with timing. He pinpointed the exact time that grass achieved its nutritional peak. He proved that if cut a week before or a week after, it had only a fraction of its protein. " My only clue was that the hens refused to eat the older grass." This was later scientifically verified by Kohler.

Thirdly, Schnabel strongly emphasized the need for "organic" farming at a time when the term was not even used. His goal was to grow 40% protein grass. He found 45% protein grass on a well-manured farm and produced 30%–40% protein oat grass on his own property. But most farmers' soil was inadequate to produce anything greater than 10%–20% protein. Schnabel pushed for the use of eggshells, seaweed, manure, autumn leaves and recycled grass fibers to enrich the soil. If it's not in the soil, it's not in the vegetable. He understood the value of minerals and trace minerals at a time when agriculture was turning to chemicals as a solution to diminishing crop yields. "Soil fertility is like money in the bank. To prosper, a farmer must put back more than he takes out."[3]

Although he never repeated the success of the mass market distribution achieved from 1940–1945, his final legacy is the fact that young cereal

---

JAMA **Journal of the American Medical Association**

Council on Foods
ACCEPTED FOODS

THE FOLLOWING PRODUCTS HAVE BEEN ACCEPTED BY THE COUNCIL ON FOODS
OF THE AMERICAN MEDICAL ASSOCIATION AND WILL BE LISTED IN THE BOOK OF
ACCEPTED FOODS TO BE PUBLISHED.   —FRANKLIN C. BING, SECRETARY, 1939

CEROPHYL

Manufacturer.—Cerophyl Laboratories (Division of American Dairies, Inc.), Kansas City, MO
Description.—Dried, powdered mixture of young leaves of wheat, oats and barley, selected and
blended to maintain the minimum vitamin potency declared on the package label.
Manufacture.—The cereals are grown on soil fertilized to produce plants of high mineral and
vitamin content. The young rapidly growing leaves are harvested just before they joint by
machinery especially designed to prevent the leaves coming in contact with the ground after
cutting. No toxic spray materials are used. The method of cultivation precludes contamination
with weeds. The freshly harvested leaves are immediately cut into short lengths and dehydrated.
Hot flue gas of minimum oxygen content is drawn from a gas furnace through the drying chamber
at an initial temperature of between approximately 800 and 900 C. The high initial temperature,
which is quickly reduced the evaporation of moisture from the grass, serves as a flash
pasteurization of the surface of the leaves. The entire process of drying requires approximately
sixty seconds. The dried material leaves the dryer at a temperature of approximately 120C. The
dehydrated leaves are mechanically cleaned, pulverized, stored at -18C. And packed in
hermetically sealed cans under nitrogen.

grasses of oats, barley, wheat and rye continue to be cut at the jointing
stage and sold as nutritional supplements, seventy years after his discovery. All of the cereal grass producers in existence today were, either directly or indirectly, spawned by the efforts of Dr. Charles F. Schnabel.

> *The new way to feed people is to grow and process 40% protein
> grass. Grass is the cheapest commercial source of vitamins and
> minerals in the world for either man or animals. High protein
> grass production will build up the land faster and at the same
> time pay larger net profits than any other crop that can be
> grown. Hunger need not be. A way has been found to banish
> starvation from the earth. It can be done with a fraction of the
> land in cultivation. No new frontiers are needed. Every nation
> now can produce the food it needs.* [4, 5] —Charles F. Schnabel

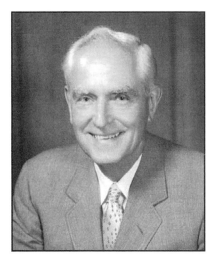

V.E. Irons

In 1900 the U.S. was in first place as far as health is concerned out of a total of 93 civilized nations. In 1920, we were in 2nd place. In 1978, we had dropped to 79th place. More than 1 notch per year. Think of it, the richest nation in wealth, knowledge, hospitals, doctors and nurses, yet near the bottom in health—all in 82 years. Yet, in 1920, we had no vitamins. A vitamin means–a live amino acid. Today the vitamin business is a (multi) billion dollar industry and our health has steadily worsened. So what good are dead vitamins? Think it over! Only LIFE begets LIFE! Only LIFE supports LIFE and only live vitamins will save us. Such is GreenLife. —V.E. Irons

V. Earl Irons was born in 1895 and grew to become one of the original pioneers of the natural foods industry. He is most famous for his belief in bowel cleansing and was first to use psyllium seed and bentonite as intestinal cleansing agents. The company he founded in 1946, still manufactures his Sonné's, Vit-Ra-Tox and Springreen cleansing products. Like many of the heroes discussed in this chapter, Irons suffered a debilitating disease that changed his life. At age 40, he was stricken with a severe arthritic disease known as ankylosing spondylitis. In desperation, he turned to natural solutions. He attributed his regime of detoxification with the successful restoration of his health and proceeded to promote these principles for the rest of his life.

Irons was no farm boy. He graduated from Yale in 1919 and lived in Boston most of his life. But Dr. Royal Lee, the founder of the famous Standard Process supplement company, brought Irons to Kansas City and introduced him to the wondrous nutritional and detoxifying benefits of grass. He started out by buying grass tablets and powder from Cerophyl and added them to his line of intestinal cleansers which he established in 1946. Impressed with the power of grass foods, he opened an office in the very same building in Kansas City where Cerophyl was headquartered

and Schnabel and Kohler worked. Eventually, he bought out one of
Schnabel's former farms and started growing and packaging his own cereal grass products. He named it *GreenLife*.

Irons vacuum dried his grass juice into powder at a low temperature
to avoid the use of any "carrier" additives. He believed in the "juice"
powder instead of dehydrated whole grass because the cellulose is indigestible. "We don't have two stomachs like cows." After beating a debilitating mid-life disease, Irons ended up starting a second family at the age
of 72, fathered his last child at 80, and at 86, moved his entire grass farm
which included the equivalent of 114 freight cars worth of tractors, trucks
and equipment. He died in 1993, just before his 99th birthday. His company, one of the oldest in the nutrition industry, still has offices in Kansas
City and is the oldest existing grass products producer in the world. *(See:
Companies)*

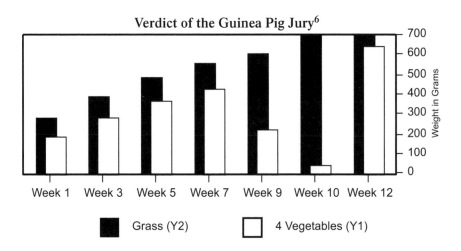

*[6]Notice that even when four of our best vegetables (spinach,
carrot, cabbage and lettuce) were fed the guinea pigs, the
growth was erratic and the pigs started to fail rapidly after the
seventh week. To save his life, dehydrated cereal grass was
added to his diet (11th week) and in less than a week, the trend
was reversed and a consistent and rapid growth took place.
The experiments prove conclusively that while other foods are
good, the grasses alone are the complete food and contain all
the elements needed to support life.   —V.E. Irons*

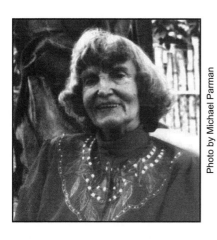

Photo by Michael Parman

The Story of Ann Wigmore

I see a world without sickness...a world in complete harmony and in perfect physical mental, and spiritual balance by following nature's laws of cause and effect.

—Ann Wigmore

Despite our historic love affair with grains and the worldwide abundance of grasses, no culture has ever cultivated the drinking of grass juice until the latter half of the twentieth century. The popular consumption of fresh squeezed wheatgrass juice is due largely to the efforts and genius of one woman, Ann Wigmore.

Sickness and Adversity Lead to Innovation

Born in Lithuania in 1909, Ann Wigmore had a rough beginning. She started out being born prematurely. Then she was abandoned because she was a sickly baby and a burden to her parents who were seeking a new life in America. Her grandmother, a self-taught naturalist, rescued and restored Ann to normal health. She learned a lot about healing by watching her grandmother heal wounded WWI soldiers with herbs and weeds. But at age 16, she still had no schooling and couldn't even write her name! At the urging of her grandmother, she left for America to get a proper education and reunite with her estranged parents. She wanted to do well in America and adopted the American lifestyle, including a typical American diet. Then a terrible automobile accident shattered both her legs. Gangrene set in and the doctors recommended amputation. She refused and even against her own father's wishes, was sent home. "My homecoming was not a happy one. Neither my father nor my mother would come near me, and only with the help of my uncle would I find something for breakfast."[7]

Ann knew there was a better way. She returned to her previous "peasant" diet of vegetables, grains, seeds and greens and restored her health by doing what she saw her grandmother do. She picked wild weeds and greens and applied them to her feet. This was not the desperation of a diseased mind, but the result of her grandmother's teaching about the healing powers of grasses and weeds. Ann developed a ravenous appetite for anything green. She nibbled on grass and sucked out its juice. She sat for hours in the warm summer sun watching the greenish-blue ring, the "creeping death" rise up her legs. Winter was approaching. There would be no more fresh grass. What to do?

I asked God for direction. He supplied an exciting solution. The use of grains to grow greens right in the kitchen!

One day to her surprise, the little white dog who gave her so much needed love and affection, started to lick her legs. This was the one part of her body he never touched! "My first thought was for the animal's safety. I impulsively raised my arm to move it away, when the injunction of my grandmother came to mind: 'Instinct-guided creatures, left to themselves, do not make mistakes.'"

That puppy was the first indicator of Ann's recovery. Rest, sun, wild herbs, weeds and kitchen–grown grasses rejuvenated Ann's health. She knew she was not going to die. The doctors informed her father that she was apparently out of danger. "This infuriated him, because he couldn't accept that he was wrong in his decision to have my feet removed." It was several months before her feet were completely healed and she returned to the hospital for an examination. The doctors "made no comment when X-ray films showed that the bones had knitted firmly," said Ann. Years later, Ann Wigmore ran in the Boston Marathon.

Ann tested her indoor grasses on her animal friends. Wheat became her favorite grass because the animals chewed more of it and it was sweet tasting, easy-to-find and inexpensive. To further her studies, she even adopted a sick, cancerous monkey. Ann nursed the monkey back to good health with creative techniques and live food recipes including: sprouted seeds, fermented nut and seed "yoghurt," and rejuvelac, a cultured sprouted wheat drink. These, along with wheatgrass, would later become the cornerstone of her Living Foods Diet.

Though she knew she had stumbled onto something very valuable, she had no practical way of making it widely available. Most people would not eat their front lawn no matter how sick they were! There had to be a better way. Then, at a local yard sale, Ann picked up an old cast iron meat grinder on the chance that it might grind the grass. With small modifications, such as the addition of a stainless steel straining sieve, this grinder became the first wheat grass juicer. It was a real innovation because commercial vegetable juicers could not at all manage the ligneous fiber of grass. This made possible her program whereby anyone could grow grass in their kitchens and extract the juice in their homes.

Ann began delivering fresh wheatgrass juice to bedridden, ill and elderly people in her Boston neighborhood. Then in 1958, she turned an old mansion on Commonwealth Avenue in Boston into The *Hippocrates Health Institute*. It was founded on the oft repeated principle of Hippocrates, the Greek father of modern medicine, who along with his hippocratic oath, is often paraphrased as saying: "The body heals itself. The physician is only nature's assistant." Dr. Ann, as she was fondly called after she became a doctor of Divinity, believed that the body can act as its own physician given the proper tools—living foods. "Living foods for living bodies, dead foods for dead bodies," said Ann.

Although Dr. Ann was neither a marketer nor a scientist, Hippocrates Health Institute, situated in the heart of Boston, attracted many celebrities and researchers who helped give testimony to the healing powers of grass. Among these were Dr. Chiu-Nan Lai, Dr G. H. Earp Thomas, Renee Taylor, Dennis Weaver, and Dick Gregory. Even Yoko Ono purchased wheatgrass for juicing in her home. People came from all walks of life and all corners of the world, usually as a "last resort," with the hopes of beating cancer or some other degenerative disease.

> *Vibrating with health and vitality, Ann Wigmore is constantly on the run. Reaching out to all that are open to hear what she has to say, she emphasizes that anyone can live a healthier, happier and more fulfilling life.*—Dennis Weaver, actor, 1984.[8]

Ann had two visitors who were enormously helpful in promoting her work. One was Viktoras Kulvinskas (see p. 35), who helped Ann establish the Hippocrates Health Living Foods program, and the other was Eydie Mae Hunsberger. Eydie had breast cancer. Her surgeon told her "You have an 80% chance to live one year and a maximum life expectancy of five years." Eydie chose a lumpectomy that removed the cancerous tissue, but it had spread. Depressed and frightened, she looked everywhere. She ended up at Dr. Ann's door in 1973. After two weeks on Dr. Ann's Living

Foods Program, Eydie was confident she would beat cancer. Two years later, with no trace of cancer in her body, she wrote *"How I conquered Cancer Naturally"*[9] which was very successful and brought many people to Dr. Ann's door.

Dr. Ann has a long list of stories and testimonials from guests who improved their health with the help of wheatgrass. Wheatgrass and its sister triticum barley, have by testimony, helped guests with ailments like high blood pressure, diabetes, obesity, gastritis, stomach ulcers, pancreas and liver troubles, asthma, glaucoma, eczema, skin problems, constipation, hemorrhoids, diverticulitis, colitis, fatigue, female problems, arthritis, athlete's foot, anemia, bad breath/body odor, and burns. In addition, wheat grass has served as a wonderful first aid for red eyes, wax in ears, congested nasal passages, bleeding gums, tooth pain, sore throats, and inflamed mucous membranes.[10, 11]

Ann tried to tell the U.S. government about wheatgrass. She even went to Washington. But the political and nutritional climate of the 1970s were stubbornly closed-minded. She had a much better reception abroad. Ann visited some twenty countries and launched living foods programs in India, Sweden, Finland and Canada. Ann learned that sickness disregarded all borders.

Let us make a concerted effort to remedy the global problems by correcting the physical and mental imbalance in each of our lives...The industrialization of our society has created an artificial lifestyle in which humans are being led further and further from the basic truths inherent in nature.[12]

In February of 1994, Ann Wigmore died of smoke inhalation in a middle of the night fire that destroyed the Boston home of the original Hippocrates Institute. She was nearly 85. Although she has passed, her work continues through the efforts of the many lives she touched. Her single clinic in Boston now has offsprings in six locations in the USA alone and others in Australia, Sweden, Finland and India. Her teachings changed the lives of millions. *(See Epilogue, In Memoriam.)*

My life has been, and continues to be, dedicated to the wellness of all humanity. —Ann Wigmore, 1909–1994

Viktoras Kulvinskas

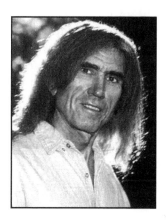

Wheatgrass juice is the nectar of rejuvenation, the plasma of youth, the blood of all life. The elements that are missing in your body's cells—especially enzymes, vitamins, hormones, and nucleic acids can be obtained through this daily green sunlight transfusion.

—Rev. Viktoras Kulvinskas

He arrived from the Massachusetts Institute of Technology. He was a mathematician and computer consultant at Harvard University. He was young, but not well. He started making some of the hard choices many of us are never able to make. He took his health in his own hands. He quit the University; turned his back on a successful career and all the security that came with it. He walked into Dr. Ann's mansion, resurrected his health and in the process became a "Gabriel" for Dr. Ann and an archangel for the living foods movement.

Viktoras was a marketing bonanza for Dr. Ann's teachings. He was the best missionary anyone could wish. In his second year there, he took Dr. Ann's book, which at the time was a magazine entitled *Be Your Own Doctor*, on a Shiloh Farms delivery truck and showed it to seventy health food stores. His "gorilla" marketing doubled her clinic's attendance from 3–6 to 6–12 students. Later, he came out with his best selling new age manual, *Survival in the 21st Century*. That inspired work, an amalgam of art, poetry, spirituality, nutrition, and gardening, served to inspire a whole generation. It quickly became a classic. This author was one of the "children" transfixed by its spell. Truly a 1970s book, it fit right in with the "tune in, turn on, and drop out" theme of the era. Only, it had nothing to do with drugs and everything to do with personal and planetary healing. It was rebellious against the S.A.D. (Standard American Diet) without any words of malice. It condemned M.D. (Medical Dogma) without harshness or anger. And it all came from a very "grass roots" (no pun intended) printing effort. The love and strength of his message quickly developed a following and Viktoras became an apostle of the new age.

Survival Into the 21st Century was also one of the first successes of the small press. Viktoras called his publishing company O'Mango'd Press. This name illustrates Viktoras' creativity and joyful spirit. It can be interpreted as being either about mangos or Man/God. The first interpretation is perfectly suited for a raw foodist press; the second is ideal for a spiritual philosophical press. His press is both, and in this one moniker he articulates the dual theme of his work.

Today, Viktoras lives in beautiful Hot Springs, Arkansas. As this book goes to press, he is in his fifty–eighth year and still taking on major projects including the new *All Life Sanctuary* retreat center *(See Resources)*. He still grows wheatgrass and still believes in raw, chlorophyll rich foods. He is a key promoter for the use of blue-green algae, another super-chlorophyll rich food. On a typical day, Viktoras works longer, sleeps fewer hours and tires less than his younger colleagues.

If only they knew, the use of grass is the most revolutionary concept introduced into the diet of society...In therapeutic amounts, wheatgrass internalizes a maximum of green chlorophyl and enzyme rich liquid food, to detoxify the body by increasing the elimination of hardened mucus, crystallized acids and solidified, decaying fecal matter. Its high enzyme content helps to dissolve tumors. It is the fastest surest way to eliminate internal waste and provide an optimum nutritional environment, so that the cosmic cell consciousness can rebuild your body.

—Rev. Viktoras Kulvinskas, MS., Survival Into the 21st Century

Yoshihide Hagiwara

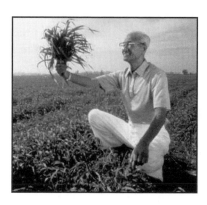

It was clear to me...that the leaves of the cereal grasses provide the nearest thing this planet offers to the perfect food...It is my belief that the steady depletion of that natural green power in the human diet, and its displacement by other nutrients of questionable value, constitutes the most serious threat of all to good health. —Yoshihide Hagiwara

About the same time Ann Wigmore was experimenting with wheatgrass juice, a pharmacist and medical doctor on the other side of the world started exploring the use of barley grass. Both barley and wheat are members of the triticum grain family. They are brother and sister seeds. It takes a close look to tell them apart. It is easier to see the differences between Wigmore and Hagiwara. Their nationalities and cultural backgrounds would be enough. But Wigmore had no marketing, science, business or financial background. Hagiwara excelled in all of these. In spite of these differences, there were some dramatic commonalities. Both had troubled childhoods and dramatic health crises. But most importantly, both were fervent believers in the power of grass.

Yoshihide Hagiwara got off to a tough start. His parents were unable to care for him and gave him away, just like Wigmore. And when his foster-mother developed cancer, she put him in an orphanage. Nevertheless, young Hagiwara had the courage and strength of character to step out on his own. He joined the Naval Academy and after he was discharged, enrolled in the University to study pharmacology. Upon graduating in 1949, he opened up a pharmacy and started inventing different formulas for his customers and neighbors, including preparations for the skin, feet and hair. Some of these are still sold in Japan today. Later, he would go back to school, this time to become a Doctor of Medicine.

In 1952, he moved to Osaka and opened a drug manufacturing company named Yamashiro Pharmaceutical Co. Ltd. There he developed and patented over 200 medications and amassed a staff of over 700. He had created the largest drug company in Japan! Hagiwara loved doing research so much, he never stopped working in the lab. But long hours, bad eating and sleeping habits, stress, and working with dangerous chemicals such as mercury, took its toll on his health. At age 38, his hair turned gray, his teeth fell out, his mind clouded up and he could no longer manage a large company. He was forced into bankruptcy.

Hagiwara, ever the fighter, mustered the strength to resurrect his health. Like Ann Wigmore, he was influenced by Hippocrates—"A disease is to be cured by man's own powers." He also studied Shin-Huang-ti, the ancient Eastern physician who compiled the fundamentals of Chinese medicine. He made a determined effort and completely transformed his diet using many Chinese herbs and fresh greens. His health returned and once again he turned his energies to finding similar solutions for others. "I began a personal search for a food which would promote good health by vitalizing the body's own power of healing."

Hagiwara's unique position was that he had the business acumen, resources and mettle to deliver a pioneering product to the modern marketplace. He was a doctor, a pharmacist, an inventor, and an experienced businessman. Perhaps the secret to Hagiwara's success, and in striking contrast to Wigmore, is that he knew in order for a product to succeed, it had to be palatable and convenient to use.

To fit into the modern world, it had to be easy to purchase, easy to use, and stable over a long period of time....What I wanted was something with a modern look and form, an ideal 'fast food.'[13]

While Wigmore's approach was to stimulate people to "be their own doctor," and grow their own food, Hagiwara wanted to give them a "fast food." His dream was to make the healing powers of green vegetables as easy to have as instant coffee. He believed that the juice of green vegetables was the finest source of nutrition. Ever the scientist, he analyzed 150 edible green plants including chickweeds, asters, pigweeds, clovers, kudzu, peas and acacias. And just like Charles Schnabel and George Kohler before him, he found that cereal grasses—barley, rye, wheat, and oats—had the most remarkable quantities of active ingredients.

Even before he turned his efforts exclusively to barley grass, Hagiwara was testing drying equipment on herbal teas. He figured if he could dehydrate Chinese herbal tea and maintain the medicinal benefits, then consumers could use these wonderful herbs as easily as they have instant coffee. Hagiwara the inventor successfully developed and patented a spray dryer that in only three seconds turned Chinese herbal tea into powder. He borrowed money from his family and friends and in 1971 established Japan Natural Foods Co. Ltd. They started out marketing high quality, powdered Chinese herbs.

Hagiwara wanted to make the benefits of green foods as easy to get as instant coffee.

Next, he turned his efforts to the cereal grasses but things didn't go smoothly. Customers were not getting results. He realized that while coffee is spray dried at 130°F, which adds a roasted aroma, this was too hot for the active ingredients in barley leaves. He refined the technique to dry at room temperatures, but the product turned brown. There were also problems with the harvesting and growing. It turned brown just sitting in the truck! He tried freezing the leaves, but that inactivated the medicinal ingredients. Like V.E. Irons in 1951, Hagiwara realized the best solution was the most expensive one—build the production facility near the fields. Although this raised production costs, he was undaunted. He was driven to perfect the product at any cost and refused to compromise. He knew that the plants needed to be harvested when they were only 8 to 10 inches tall since that is when they contain the maximum amounts of active medicinal ingredients. But this reduced the crop yield by one third over harvesting at 16–18 inches. Through trial and tribulation, Hagiwara ultimately achieved a dried barley green juice powder that maintained the nutritional integrity of the fresh plant.

In 1980, ten years after its introduction in Japan, Hagiwara brought his green barley leaf powder to the USA. In 1990, he made a major investment in American health and opened a $21 million dollar growing and processing facility in California. Hagiwara is the best kind of entrepreneur—one who puts his profits back into research. In 1981, he established the *Hagiwara Institute of Health*, which is today, the major source of nutritional information about the medicinal properties of grasses. Dr. Hagiwara's son, Hideaki Hagiwara Ph.D carrying on his father's love of science, is its director. Numerous scientific studies evaluating the medicinal properties of barley leaf juice extract have been completed in concert with scientists at the University of Tokyo, the University of California at

Davis and George Washington University, Washington DC. *(See chapter: Research)*. This research of grasses in relation to human health and nutrition is the most extensive to date and arguably is the most important legacy Yoshihide Hagiwara leaves to us.

> *What I am suggesting is that these medical tools have had the unfortunate effect of corrupting attitudes toward health. This has gone so far, I fear that now many people believe in medical and technological guarantees of good health, while little by little they give up their personal responsibility for the good health of their bodies.*[14] —Yoshihide Hagiwara

In 1994, Japan's Minister of Health and Welfare awarded Yoshihide Hagiwara the Drug and Medical Meritorious Service Award for his development of the extraction techniques used to manufacture botanical products for people and pets. While Hagiwara is clearly a pioneer in the natural foods industry, he should also be recognized for bridging the world of conventional medicine and pharmacology with natural products. He delivers scientific respect, recognition and credibility to the world of natural foods that few others have accomplished.

Accomplishments of Yoshihide Hagiwara

Inventor, Pharmacist, Entrepreneur, Medical Doctor. Founded, established and achieved the following in his lifetime:

1949   Founded Hagiwara Pharmacy
1952   Yamashiro Pharmaceutical Co., Ltd.
1968   Japan Pharmaceutical Development Co., Ltd.
1969   Hagiwara Physical and Chemical Laboratory
1971   Japan Natural Foods Co., Ltd.
1976   Green and Health Association
1978   Vice Pres. of Institute of Manufacturing all Chinese Medicine, a national institute for manufacturers.
1979   Director of Research Institute of Health Foods of Japan.
1980   Counselor of the Institute of Drugs of Osaka.
1981   Counselor, Association of Medicine Manufacturing Industry of Japan.
1981   Hagiwara Institute of Health for cancer research.
1987   Award from Japan's Science and Technology Agency.
1994   Drug and Medical Meritorious Service Award presented by Japan's Minister of Health.

Nutrition

Grass does many things in animal nutrition which cannot be accounted for by its known vitamin content.
—Dr. Charles F. Schnabel

Grass Is More than the Sum of its Parts

The vitamin supplement industry is booming. Consumers are anxious to take nutritional products as an alternative to drugs. This is a welcome trend, but where do supplements come from? Plants have been the source of our medicines for thousands of years *(See p. 217)*. Our modern drugs are largely synthetic replicas of nutritional factors found in plants—aspirin, penicillin, quinine, all came from nature. Since "our food is our medicine and our medicine is our food," as

Hippocrates the father of medicine is famous for saying, then it should logically follow that the best medicine is whole, natural food.

Even the earliest research of the 1930s identified the young cereal grasses as complete foods. All known nutrients were found including other unidentified ones called "grass juice factors." Guinea pigs lose weight and weaken on a diet of mixed vegetables but thrive on grasses. Mega doses of vitamin supplements can function like medicines to stimulate or enhance biological function. But nutrients don't live in a vacuum. They co-exist with numerous other factors that enhance and enable their function. Once isolated, they may not work as well. Albert Szent-Györgyi, the Nobel prize bio-chemist who discovered ascorbic acid, found that natural vitamin C was more therapeutic than the synthetic ascorbic acid even though they were chemically identical. When we start adding isolated vitamins of different kinds to our diet, it is a case of man trying to imitate nature. Nutrition by the numbers. How many milligrams of calcium in relation to magnesium, and magnesium in relation to phosphorous is the perfect balance? A whole food is a complex bundle of thousands of chemicals. Squeezing out isolated nutrient fractions dissipates its magic. Grass contains hundreds of vitamins, minerals, enzymes, amino acids, phytochemicals, anti-oxidants, immunomodulators, cellular RNA and DNA all in concentrated form. Like grass, spirulina, chlorella, blue green algae, and bee pollen are a few other wonderful natural foods containing a broad spectrum of concentrated nutrients. These foods give our bodies the raw materials from which it manufactures what it needs and balances its own chemistry. The philosophy of this book is that where basic nutrition is concerned, concentrated whole foods make the best supplements.

It is folly to dose ourselves with one or two vitamins when we know nothing of their relationships to fifty other food factors.
—Charles F. Schnabel

Nutrition Depends on Where, When and How

It all starts in the soil. The earth feeds the plants and the plants feed us. When you walk into your natural food store to purchase grass, it may have come from the high terrain of Utah, the plains of Kansas, the Pacific Coast of California, or the greenhouse of your local grower. They may all be organically grown, but they can't all be nutritionally identical. There is no equality in nature. Regardless of whether you are growing strawberries, tomatoes, or grass, the nutritional analysis will vary from state to state, grower to grower, and farm to farm. From soil, to water, to weather, disorder is the fundamental law of nature. Was the season too hot or too cold? Too wet or too dry? Growing times for grass vary from 60 days to 200 days in the field, and 10 to 14 days in the greenhouse. Some tray grass growers can eliminate a few variables with climate controlled greenhouses and automated irrigation. But processing has yet another influence. Is your grass fresh or frozen, freeze dried or spray dried? Drum dried or evaporated? At what temperature? Was the whole leaf ground and powdered or was the grass juiced and dried? What was the method of juicing? How was it bottled? In glass or plastic? Colored or clear? Nitrogen flushed? Hermetically sealed? Even two samples of grass squeezed fresh right in front of you can look and taste different. It depends on who grew it, where it was grown, what type of soil, seed, temperature, water, harvest time, etc.

Okay, there are many variables, but don't be dismayed. Grass is a food and these variables exist with every fruit and vegetable you eat. Of course, you can always grow your own. But you still won't be able to control the variables. Are you ready to invest the time and materials? Are you sure you can do a better job than the professionals? Can you be sure you will produce a nutritionally superb crop? (For more, see *The Companies* and *Grow Your Own*.)

Harvest at the Peak of Nutrition–The Jointing Theory

In 1930 Charles Schnabel fed a flock of sick chickens grass. They completely recovered and ultimately achieved phenomenal fertility. As an agricultural chemist, he was able to figure out why. The young oat grass had something special about it that wasn't in the mature grass. "My only clue was that the hens refused to eat the older grass."[1] Schnabel repeated his experiments the following summer and isolated the exact moment of its maximum nutrition. The differences in nutritional content were so remarkable, depending on the time of harvest, that Schnabel eventually received a U.S. patent for his discovery. Essentially it is this: the plant undergoes rapid growth with increasing nutritional manifestation until maturity when it switches gears from vegetative growth to reproductive growth. Just prior to this changeover, the plant is at its nutritional peak. This transition is known as jointing. Technically, it is when the ovul of grain moves up the staff from the root. It only takes a few days. After jointing, the nutritional counts drop radically. The plant then starts sending all its nour-

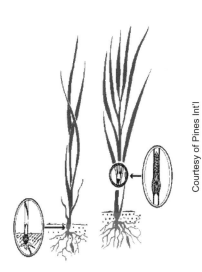

Courtesy of Pines Int'l

Think of jointing as a kind of puberty for a plant. At this stage it is primed for maximum nutrition.

ishment into the developing seed. The grass grows quickly, and starts blooming and producing grain. Although harvesting a week later would produce much more the amount per acre, the nutritional level would be dramatically inferior.

Because this discovery had tremendous influence on the livestock feed industry and secondarily on human nutrition—via their milk and meat—there was much interest in verifying it. In 1935 Phillips and Goss reported that a field of barley contained 38.8% protein on the 21st day of growth (the jointing stage), 12.2% protein on the 49th day (the bloom stage) and 3.8% protein on the 86th day (the mature stage).[3] Also that year George Kohler, the most active grass researcher of his time, reported that most of the vitamins in grass reach a peak per gram of dry matter at or near the jointing stage roughly paralleling the protein content. This peak may be twice as high on the day of jointing as it is a week before or a week after.

> *...It should be obvious that the phenomenal feeding value of good grass at the jointing stage is a transient quality. If it is not grazed or cut and preserved within a few days of the jointing stage, its value is lost forever because the vitamins associated with photosynthesis are not transferred to the grain or returned to the soil. They are used up by the grass plant during the reproductive stage of growth. It is this transient nature of grass quality at the jointing stage that has made the secret of grass so elusive. The irony of it is that our "dumb" animals seem to have known the secret all the time.*
> —Charles F. Schnabel[2]

What's So Great about Grass?

All vegetables are food factories. Each excels in different nutrient areas. Because eggs have 12% protein, meat 17%, and whole leaf grass 25%, we could define grass as a protein food. But there are other foods like algaes with higher protein than grass. Why should we even bother with the lower protein foods? Because nutrition is not a weight lifting contest. It's not about getting more protein, but more equilibrium. It's not quantity, but quality and the most important part of that is diversity and balance. Grass is a balanced food containing a broad spectrum of high quality vegetable nutrition. It is a rainbow food and at the end of the rainbow is the promise of golden health. Grass does not zoom you there with speed, but carries you there gently on the magic carpet of endurance and delivers you with strength and longevity.

What's in Grass?

- The "Grass Juice Factor"
- All Known Proteins & Peptides
- Concentrated Nutrition
- All Known Vitamins & Minerals
- Chlorophyll and Carotenoids
- Antioxidants for Detoxification
- Quick Assimilation
- Active Enzymes
- Immunomodulators
- Grow Hormones

The blade of grass contains all the elements of which the body is composed including revitalizing and rebuilding materials, force producers for energy and also the eliminators of waste acids. Grass and sprouts are perfect foods. —Dr. Ann Wigmore

Grasses are a complete life sustaining food. Based on the animal studies (see *Research*), if you had to choose one food for survival, it ought to be grass. After all, grasses are the primary food for domestic and wild grazing animals and some pretty large ones at that—cows, horses, goats, sheep, buffalo, deer, giraffes. The guinea pigs, chickens, rats and other laboratory animals were losing weight on our finest vegetables but quickly reversed their downward trends when switched to grass. (See chapters: *Pioneers, Research*.) These dumb animals have long known the truth about grass. We are just coming around now because we have the technological means to compensate for our inability to digest the grass directly. Instead of four compartments in our stomachs, we have juicing machines and micro-fine powdering equipment.

Fifteen pounds of wheat grass is equivalent to 350 pounds of the choicest vegetables. —Charles F. Schnabel

Blue-green algae, chlorella, and spirulina are wonderful and important superfoods that surpass grasses in certain nutrient categories and should be in our diet. But they are more expensive to cultivate than grasses their cost per nutrient is high. Man has evolved from the land and historically, land grown foods are best suited for land based animals. Charles Schnabel was so impressed with the inexpensive cost of vitamins from grass, he created a "Yard-Stick" for measuring the value of foods in terms of pennies per nutrient. According to Schnabel: "only one-half ounce of 40% protein dehydrated grass would supply 18,600 units of vitamin A, 113 milligrams of vitamin C, and 5.7 grams of the best quality protein in the world. This is more vitamin A than supplied by the entire 84.5 ounces of food in the (USDA recommended) optimum diet and more vitamin C than is supplied by the entire 30 ounces of fruits and vegetables."

Grass is a wonderfully balanced source of nutrients. Excellent for all minerals major and minor, it is especially high in calcium, magnesium, manganese, phosphorus, and potassium, as well as trace minerals such as zinc and selenium. All are important for cardiovascular and immune system function. Grass is a source for all B-vitamins including folic acid, pantothenic acid, an abundance of choline, and is a vegetable source of

Some of the Nutrients in Grass

Amino Acids: Tryptophan, Glutamic Acid, Alanine, Methionine, Arginine, Lysine, Aspartic Acid, Cystine, Glycine, Histidine, Isoleucine, Leucine, Phenylalanine, Proline, Serine, Threonine, Tyrosine, Valine. Small polypeptides.

Enzymes: (Over 80 have been identified) Super-oxide Dismutase, Peroxidase, Phosphatase, Catalase, Cytochrome Oxidase, DNase, RnaseSuperoxide, Hexokinase, Malic dehydrogenase, Nitrate reductase, Nitrogen oxyreductase, Fatty Acid Oxidase, Phosolipase, Polyphenoloxidase, Dismutase, Transhydrogenase.

Phytochemicals: Chlorophyll, Carotenoids, Bioflavonoids, growth hormones, RNA, DNA

Vitamins: Vitamin C, vit. E (succinate), Beta-carotene (vit.A) Biotin, Choline, Folic Acid, B1-Thiamine, B2-Riboflavin, B3-Niacin, B6-Pantothenic Acid, vit. K

Minerals & Trace Minerals: Zinc, Selenium, Phosphorus, Potassium, Calcium, Boron, Chloride, Chromium, Cobalt, Copper, Iodine, Iron, Magnesium, Manganese, Nickel, Sodium, Sulfur. (These are the primary ones, there are many more.)

Fatty Acids: Linolenic Acid, Linoleic Acid.

B-12. Fresh wheatgrass juice is 2% protein and there is up to 45% in barley grass juice powder. An egg, the symbol of fertility long considered the perfect protein, is 42% protein (dried). Protein in grass is in the form of poly-peptides—simpler, shorter chains of amino acids—that enable faster, more efficient assimilation into the bloodstream and tissues. Grass includes at least 20 amino acids both essential and non-essential. Its spectrum of vitamins is so broad, that in 1939, dehydrated wheat grass was actually accepted by the American Medical Association as a natural vitamin food. *(See p. 28)*

The Magic of Chlorophyll

Whenever anyone talks about the healing powers of grass, they mention chlorophyll first. Grasses, along with alfalfa and algaes, are the richest sources of chlorophyll on the planet. No surprise here. One third of the planet is covered with grass including even the one inch tundra above the Arctic Circle. Chlorophyll and the omnipresence of grass are essential to life on the planet. Green plant cells are the only ones capable of absorbing energy directly from the sun. The primeval energy for all life is thus light. Sunlight radiation is absorbed by plants and secondarily by humans and animals. If the energy output from the sun were to cease, the basic vital functions of all living organisms would gradually slow down, and eventually life on Earth would become extinct. It takes eight minutes for a photon of light to travel the ninety-three million miles from the sun to the Earth's surface. A green plant needs only a few seconds to capture that energy, process it, and store it in the form of a chemical—chlorophyll. This process of converting light into energy is called photosynthesis.

All forms of life, on land and in the sea, even when they feed on each other, are parasites, depending ultimately on plant life. Your body, its flesh and its organs are made up largely of protein coming to you directly from food plants or the flesh of plant eating animals. You personally, exist only because of chlorophyll. —Dr. T. M. Rudolph[4]

PHOTOSYNTHESIS CREATES LIFE

Cells in leaves do miraculous things. Water and carbon dioxide enter the leaf. Photons of visible light from sunshine are captured in cells called chloroplasts. As the chloroplasts absorb the light, their electrons become excited. They are literally dancing in the sunshine. They are charged with energy that is stored as ATP (adenosine triphosphate). The ATP then reduces carbon dioxide and water to oxygen and glucose—sugar. The oxygen exits the leaf and fills the atmosphere with fresh air and the sugar remains as food for all animal life. Were chemists able to duplicate photosynthesis by artificial means, we would be able to harness the power of the sun—solar energy—for all our energy needs.

Famous research scientist E. Bircher called chlorophyll "concentrated sun power" and reported that it "increases the functions of the heart, affects the vascular system, the intestines, the uterus, and the lungs. It raises the basic nitrogen exchange and is therefore a tonic which, considering its stimulating properties, cannot be compared with any other."[5]

One of the reasons chlorophyll is so effective is its similarity to hemin or heme. Hemin is part of "hemoglobin," the protein portion of human blood that carries oxygen. Studies as long ago as 1911 show that the molecules of hemin and chlorophyll are surprisingly alike. The primary distinction is that chlorophyll is bound by an atom of magnesium and hemin is bound by iron. Experiments prove that severely anemic rabbits make a rapid return to a normal blood count once chlorophyll is administered.[6]

Is the body able to substitute iron and rebuild the blood because of chlorophyll? We have proven that wheatgrass works for anemics and thalassemics (see *Research*). Is it because of the chlorophyll-hemin pathway?

Chlorophyll has long been famous for its ability to heal infected and ulcerated wounds. Studies prove that "tissue cell activity and its normal regrowth are definitely increased by using chlorophyll."[7] It is an important medicine for healing bleeding gums, canker sores, trench mouth, pyorrhea, gingivitis, even sore throat. Chlorophyll has the unique ability to be absorbed directly through the mucous membranes, especially those of the nose, throat, and digestive tract. It makes a great mouth wash and an excellent dentifrice, especially when used in powder

Chlorophyll
$C_{55}H_{72}MgN_4O_5$

form. Chlorophyll's unique ability to kill anaerobic–odor producing bacteria–is the reason it covers up the smell of garlic, fights bad breath, body odor, and acts as a general antiseptic. These bacteria live without air and are destroyed by chlorophyll's oxygen producing agents. Dr. Otto Warburg, the 1931 Nobel prize winner for physiology and medicine, concluded that oxygen deprivation was a major cause of cancer. At least one alternative cancer therapy today bombards tumors with ozone—highly active oxygen. Unlike many drugs, chlorophyll has never been found to be toxic at any dose. And in their natural state, none of the 9,000 species of grasses that cover our planet is poisonous.

Chlorophyll may even provide us with protection from low level X-ray radiation from hospital equipment, televisions, computer screens, transmitters, and microwaves. Radiation poisoned guinea pigs recovered when chlorophyll rich vegetables were added to their diet.[8] The U.S. Army repeated this experiment with broccoli and alfalfa and got the same results.[9]

Grass – A Cornucopia of Enzymes & Nutrients

But chlorophyll is only one of the important pigments in grass. There are other pigments such as carotenoids—alpha-carotene and the famous beta-carotene, xanthophylls, and zeaxanthin to name a few. There are an abundance of these phytonutrient pigments in grass. Unfortunately, you can't see them because as with the beautiful autumn leaves, chlorophyll overpowers the other pigments. There are up to 18,000 units of beta-carotene per ounce of grass. This pre-cursor of vitamin A has significant immune-enhancing properties including the promotion of T-cells. High levels of this anti-oxidizing nutrient are associated with reduced cancer risk and cardiovascular disease.

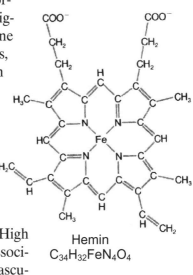

Hemin
$C_{34}H_{32}FeN_4O_4$

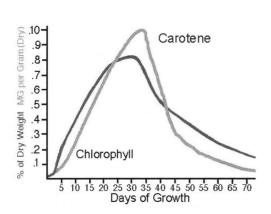

The two most important pigments in grass—chlorophyll and carotene peaking at the jointing stage.

Another important vitamin and antioxidant abundant in grass is vitamin E. Grasses have a water soluble form of E called a-tocopherol succinate that stimulates the production of T-cells, antibodies, interleukin2, and interferon among its many immune system functions. This form of vitamin E is very effective in suppressing the growth of cancer cells in vitro. In addition, it has the ability to increase production of prolactin and growth hormone in the pituitary gland. *(See p. 62)* Grasses are also abundant sources of quality vitamin K, the blood clotting vitamin. The body needs it to form the enzyme prothrombin which creates fibrin that clots blood. It also acts as an antidote for certain poisons.

Dr. T. Shibamoto of the University of California, discovered a powerful new antioxidant in barley grass called 2″-0-GIV. This new isoflavonoid is both soluble in water and fats and is highly stable. This means it is capable of permeating both the fat and aqueous cell membranes in order to fully protect the cell from the damaging effects of oxidation. According to Shibamoto, 2″-0-GIV is more potent than vitamins E and C, but when taken together, the effects are profound. Barley grass has all three in good quantity. Tests have shown it is a preventative for arteriosclerosis and is just as effective as the prescription drug Probutol for this disease, without any side effects. *(See p. 76)*

Barley and wheat grass are both abundant, inexpensive sources of superoxide dismutase (SOD). This is a powerful antioxidant and anti-aging enzyme. SOD is a proven anti-inflammatory for arthritis, edema, gout, bursitis, etc. Dr. K. Kubota of the Science University of Tokyo found two glyco-proteins D1G1 and P4D1 that work alongside SOD but are more heat stable. All three have anti-inflammatory action that is superior to the much touted aspirin.

Good grass manufacturers test SOD as a yard-stick for measuring overall enzyme activity. If the heat sensitive SOD is active, so are all the other 80+ enzymes in grass. When most people think of enzymes they think of digestive enzymes such as lactase, amylase, protease and lipase. But these do not alone digest all foods and digestion is not the only function of enzymes. DNA, found in every plant food for example, requires the enzyme Dnase for digestion. Enzymes also detoxify harmful substances and participate in thousands of never-ending chemical changes in the body. Powdered grass products are carefully processed to preserve as many enzymes as possible. Fresh squeezed wheatgrass juice is a veritable enzyme soup, its cells dancing with metabolic activity. It is so charged with "chi" or bio-electric energy, you can feel it rushing through your body or raising the hair on the back of your neck. Wheatgrass juice is liquid sunshine transformed into nutritive energy. A veritable brew of water, oxygen, enzymes, protein, phytochemicals, chlorophyll, carotenoids, fatty acids, and trace minerals are all rushing to revitalize you.

Nutrition Charts

The following nutritional charts represent comparisons between grass, vegetables and common foods. Where they are available, a variety of different grasses are represented. When you study these charts, keep in mind some of the themes expressed in the early pages of this chapter. A) Grass is more than the sum of its parts. B) Micro-managing our body chemistry—nutrition by the numbers—is not the best idea. C) Health is not measured in hundreds of milligrams, but by balance and quality. D) Nutrient amounts are in constant flux due to a range of natural variables.

Analysis of Indoor Grown Fresh Wheatgrass Juice per Ounce					
Moisture	95%	**Vitamin A**	122 IU	**Phosphorus**	21.4mg
Protein	1.9–2.8%	**Vitamin B-12**	.3mcg	**Magnesium**	8mg
Sugars	2–3%	**Vitamin E**	4.3 IU	**Iron**	.66mg
Chlorophyll	4–12mg	**Vitamin C**	1mg	**Calcium**	7.2mg
Biotin	2.86mcg	**Folic Acid**	8.3 mcg	**Potassium**	42mg

Source: Irvine Analytical Labs. Irvine, CA. Courtesy Optimum Health Institute.

Lab reports can be confusing. If you can read and understand these data charts, then this book has done its job. First of all, different labs use different units of measure even for the same things. You may find either IU–international units or mcg–micrograms for elements such as beta-carotene and vitamin E. Some use metric system terms like ML–milliliters while other use ounces and tablespoons. Some measure according to serving size while others use the 100g (gram) standard. Converting all the different lab reports to one standard measure is quite a job and beyond the ken of the average consumer. If that weren't hard enough, mainstream departments of nutrition haven't yet discovered wheatgrass and standard lab analyses don't even include chlorophyll. The numbers you see here have been derived from a variety of labs and manufacturers and is the best and latest available at the time.

Sorry, No Brands

It is not the goal of this book to provide the nutritional analyses of the various brands and compare them. These charts do not identify commercial products. So you won't be getting recommendations for Nestlés over

Hershey's or Mars. However, the charts do compare the different classes of products such as indoor vs. outdoor grown, barley vs. wheat, whole leaf vs. juice, etc. And don't forget *The Companies* chapter, where you get lots of background about the different manufacturers which will help you match your personal preferences to the products.

Chlorophyll Comparisons

The chlorophyll comparisons chart compares the chlorophyll in green foods including tray-grown fresh and freeze dried, outdoor-grown whole leaf and juice powders, and the algaes. Unfortunately, number to number comparisons of fresh squeezed juice to dried juice powder are not fair because fresh juice is 95% water. Once you remove that water, however, the solids left behind are indeed the nutritional portion of the juice. They also provide a stable platform for analysis. The numbers for fresh juice really don't do it justice. These labs mostly measure macro-nutrients—proteins, carbohydrates, minerals, vitamins, etc. But the magic of grass

Chlorophyll and Protein in Green Foods			
Units are % of total content. All grasses except 'fresh' are powders	Moisture	Protein	Chlorophyll
Fresh Wheatgrass Juice	95.0%	1.9–2.8%	0.1–0.2%
Whole Leaf Wheat Grass	7.0%	25.0%	0.6%
Kamut Wheat Grass Juice	5–9%	19–27%	0.3–0.7%
Alfalfa Juice	0.3%	38.0%	0.7–1.2%
Barley Grass Juice	6–8%	27–46%	0.5–0.6%
Freeze Dried Tray Grown	8.0%	43.0%	0.1%
Wheatgrass Juice	4–7%	32–40%	0.6–1.1%
Spirulina	4–7%	60.0%	1.0%
Chlorella	5.0%	55–65%	2–3%
Blue Green Algae	2.0%	62.0%	1–2%

Source: Compilation of various reports. All items are powders unless otherwise stated "fresh." Tray grown is indoor grown wheatgrass juice. Juice means the grass is juiced then dried. Whole leaf means the leaves are dried and powdered, not juiced.

juice, fresh or dried, lies in its micro-nutrients—the enzymes, growth factors, immunomodulators, carotenoids, small polypeptides, etc. They don't usually show up on these reports anyway.

When comparing chlorophyll counts between indoor and outdoor-grown grasses, remember the many differences between them *(see p. 92)*. There are more nutrients and plant compounds in the solids of the more mature outdoor-grown grass. Notice how the chlorophyll counts are significantly higher in the powders than in the two tray-grown products— the fresh and freeze-dried. This is partly because the outdoor grass has unobstructed exposure to solar energy and partly because of its mature roots. This represents the limitations of indoor agriculture. All the other grasses listed are outdoor-grown. Higher chlorophyll counts also indicate the quality of the growing, juicing, and drying process. Chlorophyll will degrade upon exposure to heat and oxygen. When it does, it creates a by-product called pheophorbide. High chlorophyll and low pheophorbide suggests good care was taken from farming through processing.

Moisture figures are included in this chart because they have a significant relationship with all other nutrient counts. As you can see, the tray-grown fresh wheatgrass juice is 95% water and about 2% protein. If you remove the water, as was done in the "freeze-dried tray grown," it would be about 40% protein. The more moisture there is, the lower the nutrient numbers. Ranges are given wherever multiple analyses were obtained and they remind us about the numerous agricultural variations.

The Seventy Percent Chlorophyll Myth

There is a common misconception from the 1970s that fresh wheatgrass juice contains 70% chlorophyll. In fact, it is only about one-tenth of one percent chlorophyll. How could this be? For starters, fresh juice is 95% water. The solid content of the juice, the essence of its nutrition, makes up approximately 5%. Of that, 2% is protein and another 2% is sugar. For comparison, carrot juice is 89% water, 4% sugar, and 1% protein. Apple juice is 88% water, 11% sugar and has no significant protein. The protein in wheatgrass actually includes a full range of amino acids, enzymes, and small polypeptides. In the remaining 1% of its "essence" lies over 100 other nutrients, growth factors, immunomodulators, plant hormones, and as yet unnamed "grass juice factors." Even outdoor-grown wheatgrass with its broad solar collector leaves has about 0.5% chlorophyll (543mg per 100 grams) for the whole-leaf powder. Outdoor-grown grass juice powder ranges between 0.7% and 1.2%chlorophyll. Even the algaes, the world's most chlorophyll-rich foods, only fall in the 2% range. Basically, this green pigment, responsible for capturing sunlight, does not comprise a large percentage of any green plant. However, the grasses, along with alfalfa and the algaes, are our finest sources of it. Chlorophyll still performs its miracles even at this low dosage. But keep in mind that chlorophyll is only one of many of potent therapeutic factors in grass.

Acknowledgments

The grasses used in these analyses are tray-grown fresh squeezed wheatgrass juice, tray-grown freeze-dried wheatgrass juice, whole leaf dehydrated grass, wheat and barley grass juice powders, Kamut juice powder and carbon dioxide dried wheatgrass juice powder. All data is reported by certified laboratories. The analyses were provided courtesy of Pines International, Green Foods Corp. Green Kamut Corp., Sheldon Farms, Synergy Productions, VitaRich Foods, The Optimum Health Institute, V.E. Irons, Inc., and U.S. Dept. of Agriculture Human Nutrition Research Center. A special thanks is given to these organizations. To find out more about these sources see: *The Companies, Wheatgrass Retreats*, and *The Pioneers*.

The Many Variables of Lab Reports

Variation is the underlying theme when evaluating lab reports. Even within one company and for one product, nutrient counts can vary dramatically from season to season and report to report. Even if the very same batch is brought into two certified laboratories, it brings different results. We tend to think that science is immutable. But testing equipment and environments differ and this natural product, especially when fresh, changes molecule by molecule and minute by minute. With incubation times as long as 20 hours for some tests, it is a race to quantify nutrients before they perish. Don't read too much into these numbers. The best we can do is look at averages. Of course you want the best. Just choose the type of grass you prefer, and go with a reputable brand in which you have faith.

Vitamin & Mineral Comparison of Grass & Common Foods							
per 100 grams		Grass	Sprouts	Spinach	Broccoli	Eggs	Chicken
Protein	g	25	7.490	2.860	2.980	12.440	17.550
Fat	g	7.980	1.270	.350	.350	9.980	20.330
Calcium	mg	321.000	28.000	99.000	48.000	49.000	10.000
Iron	mg	24.900	2.140	2.710	.880	1.440	1.040
Magnesium	mg	112.000	82.000	79.000	25.000	10.000	20.000
Phosphorus	mg	575.000	200.000	49.000	66.000	177.000	172.000
Potassium	mg	3,225.000	169.000	558.000	325.000	120.000	204.000
Sodium	mg	18.800	16.000	79.000	27.000	280.000	71.000
Zinc	mg	4.870	1.650	.530	.400	1.100	1.190
Copper	mg	0.375	.261	.130	.045	.014	.074
Manganese	mg	2.450	1.858	.897	.229	.026	.019
Selenium	mcg	2.500	n/a	1.000	3.000	30.800	n/a
Vitamin C	mg	214.500	2.600	28.100	93.200	0.000	2.400
Thiamin	mg	0.350	.225	.078	.065	.049	.114
Riboflavin	mg	16.900	.155	.189	.119	.430	.167
Niacin	mg	8.350	3.087	.724	.638	.062	6.262
Pantothenic	mg	0.750	.947	.065	.535	1.125	.920
Vitamin B-6	mg	1.400	.265	.195	.159	.118	.330
Folate	mcg	1,110.000	38.000	194.400	71.000	35.000	6.000
Vit. B-12	mcg	0.800	0.000	0.000	0.000	.800	.320
Vitamin A	IU	513.000	0.000	6715.00	n/a	632.000	178.000
Vit A, RE	mcg	2,520.000	0.000	672.000	154.000	190.000	52.000
Vitamin E	mg	9.100	.050	1.890	1.660	1.050	n/a

Data compiled from USDA Nutrient Data Laboratory Release 11-1, whole leaf dehydrated wheat grass from Pines International (Southern Testing & Research Laboratories). Sprouts are three day old wheat sprouts.

Key Nutrients in Different Dried Grasses

	Wheat Grass Juice Powder	Whole Leaf Wheat grass	Freeze Dried Wheatgrass Juice	Kamut Wheat Grass Juice	Barley Grass Juice
Phos	n/a	575	2,700	249	594
Mag	380	112	400	n/a	225
Calc	630	321	450	1,110	718
Potas	6,100	3,225	250	4,970	2,762
Beta-C	34,900	15,230	4,140	8,940	39,680
Vit E	5.73	12	2.2	7.24	16.2
Vit B-12	5.24	2.38	10.00	n/a	n/a
Vit C	235	215	17	113	132
Iron	25	25	n/a	n/a	16
Zinc	3	5	6	4	7

Phosphorus, Magnesium, Calcium, Potassium, Beta-Carotene. All units in mg/100grams except for int'l units (IU) for Beta-Carotene and Vitamin E, and micrograms (mcg) for Vitamin B-12. Compilation from various reports. See acknowledgments.

8 Essential Amino Acids of Grass & Common Foods

per 100 grams		Grass	Sprouts	Spinach	Broccoli	Eggs	Chicken
Threonine	g	1.360	.254	.122	.091	.597	.726
Isoleucine	g	1.450	.287	.147	.109	.679	.877
Phenylalanine	g	1.820	.350	.129	.084	.661	.682
Arginine	g	2.030	.425	.162	.145	.746	1.099
Alanine	g	2.280	.295	.142	.118	.693	1.021
Aspartic acid	g	4.310	.453	.240	.213	1.250	1.565
Glutamic acid	g	4.350	1.871	.343	.375	1.626	2.568
Proline	g	1.570	.674	.112	.114	.496	.846

Wheatgrass used is indoor grown freeze dried 42.8% protein, 8.4% moisture, courtesy of Sheldon Farms (analysis by Northeast Labs.) Sprouts are 3 day old wheat sprouts. Vegetable data from USDA Human Nutrition Research Center Nutrient Data Lab Release 11-1.

Soil vs. Non-Soil

One of the many controversies in the wheatgrass world is the question of whether growing grass hydroponically is good enough. We have addressed this question in our gardening discussion (see p. 57) and took the position that for indoor gardening, wheatgrass is virtually just as potent whether you grow it in soil or in water. Of course, adding liquid kelp or other mineral products to that water enhances your results. Here we have an actual lab analysis so you can see for yourself. Two trays were grown in the same greenhouse under the same conditions using the same seed. One used composted organic soil, the other just water. According to Mr. John Howell, of the Soil Lab at the University of Mass. Extension, the two products are virtually equal: "It appears as though the grass has not begun to get nutrients from the composted soil but is still growing off the initial nutrient base of the seed."

Wheatgrass—Soil vs. Non-Soil			
Nutritional comparison of wheatgrass grown in organic composted soil and in water using the same seed			
Element	**Water**	**Soil**	**Differences**
Nitrogen (N)	5.92%	5.82%	Not significant
Phosphorus (P)	0.65%	0.63%	No difference
Potassium (K)	1.03%	1.17%	Not significant
Calcium (CA)	0.22%	0.30%	Not significant
Magnesium (MG)	0.14%	0.17%	No difference
Zinc (ZN)	44ppm	47ppm	No difference
Copper (CU)	15ppm	14ppm	No difference
Manganese (MN)	23ppm	24ppm	No difference
Iron (FE)	87ppm	108ppm	Not significant
Boron (B)	1ppm	2ppm	Not significant
Molybdenum (MO)	1ppm	1ppm	No difference

Test results courtesy of Jonathan's Organic Sprouts, Marion, Mass. www.jonathansorganic.com

Supplements vs. Whole Food Concentrates

If you want an always dependable milligram amount for a specific nutrient, then buy supplements. But the disadvantage of supplements is that they are usually isolated nutrients or man-made formulas. Although they have many benefits, the advantage of grasses and other superfoods is they are nature-made whole food concentrates, not man-made nutrient combinations. The dosages in whole foods may not be as high as your vitamin supplements, but they are significant nonetheless. Whole foods have a qualitative advantage because they are naturally synergistic. This enhances the bio-activity of their nutrients, increases assimilation, and provides therapeutic benefit even at low dosage.

One of the themes of this book is the rejection of nutrition by the numbers. These lab reports show that there is much nutrition in powdered grass, but it is harder to pinpoint the nutrition in fresh juice. Fresh products are simply less stable and yet it should be your goal to eat more fresh, organic foods. It's as if the fresh juice refuses to allow its magic to be quantified. Processing and powdering is not a perfect world, but it is convenient. The trade-off for bottled grass is time and effort. You don't have to clean your juicer or wash your vegetables or shop for organic produce or grow anything. That has its value.

While the nutrition information in this chapter is important, the people who have been drinking wheatgrass juice for decades don't need nutrient analyses. They take wheatgrass on faith. For more on why wheatgrass has value beyond its nutrition, see *Science & Wheatgrass.*

Only by understanding the wisdom of natural foods and their effects on the body shall we attain the mastery of disease and pain. —William Harvey, 1578–1657. English physician who discovered circulation of the blood and the role of the heart.

Research

The power of wheatgrass is extraordinary. It never ceases to amaze me. Yes, it's begging for formal proof. But the results are self-evident. Not everything needs a double blind trial. It's safe. It's a food. If you've got someone with a burn and in pain and you can stop the pain, seal off the wound, prevent infection, and heal it without scarring overnight...why would you need a double blind study to use it?

—Dr. C.L. Reynolds, M.B., B.S., Melbourne, Australia

Nutritional advances are usually developed by isolating nutritional factors and assessing their benefits to human health. These can be the macro-nutrients—vitamins, minerals, proteins, fats, and carbohydrates. But more often they are the micro-nutrients—enzymes, flavonoids, carotenoids, fatty acids, small peptides, bioflavonoids, immunomodulators, plant hormones, and antioxidants. Some factors cannot be isolated and therefore remain unnamed until they can be identified and characterized. Such is the case when you read about "the grass juice factor," first proposed in the 1930s. Grass still contains secret micro-nutrients that escape our classification even today.

There was a flurry of studies on cereal grasses and their healing properties in the 1930s and 1940s thanks largely to the efforts of Charles Schnabel. After that there were many dry years until Yoshihide Hagiwara came along. As a medical doctor and pharmacist, Hagiwara matched his considerable business skills with his talents as a researcher. His contribution to the science behind the healing powers of young green cereal grasses, and barley grass in particular, is enormous and we have all benefitted from his lifelong contribution. His passing in 2004 marked the end of an era for the entire grass industry. Barley grass dominates the research in this chapter because of Hagiwara's prodigious work. But barley, wheat, oats, Kamut, and rye are all brother and sister triticums. Many claim that barley is the superior grass. You can make your own decisions about which grass is best for you. This book, despite its title, embraces all grasses with equal enthusiasm.

Some Benefits of Grass Substantiated by Research

- Repairs DNA
- Enhances Immunity
- Stops Free-Radicals
- Inhibits Carcinogens
- Increases Longevity
- Provides Growth Hormone
- Helps Skin Diseases
- Reduces Cholesterol
- Prevents Inflammation
- Promotes Cellular Rejuvenation
- Enhances Stamina & Endurance
- Neutralizes Pesticides
- Provides Antioxidants
- Lowers Atherosclerosis Risk

Some of the studies in this chapter were carried out on animals such as rats, guinea pigs, chicks, rabbits, or hamsters. Some are epidemiological studies that map trends on populations and groups. Others test substances in the laboratory (in vitro) against other materials including human cells and blood. The ultimate test is a human study (in vivo) where real people are tested as they take the product. To learn more about the relationship between science and wheatgrass as well as *How to Study a Study*, see the chapter: *Science & Wheatgrass*.

Growth Stimulating Factor and Complete Food

The Relation of the Grass JuiceFactor to Guinea Pig Nutrition. By G.O. Kohler, C.A. Elvehjem, and E.B. Hart, Department of Agriculture Chemistry, University of Wisconsin, Madison, Pub November 24, 1937 in the Journal of Nutrition, Vol.15, p. 445. No.5. Also, The Grass Juice Factor, by G. Kohler, S. Randle, and J. Wagner. Journal of Biology and Chemistry. V.128. 1939.

Research into the nutritional content of cereal grasses and curiosity about their secret health-promoting factors began in the USA in 1935. A group of scientists from the Department of Agricultural Chemistry at the University of Wisconsin ran a series of experiments in an attempt to learn why milk produced by cows in the winter on winter rations was markedly inferior to milk produced by cows grazing in the spring and summer on fresh pastures. They began adding grass powder to the winter feed and monitored the results on guinea pigs since they, like cows, are herbivorous animals. They concluded that "the growth stimulating factor of grass was distinct from all the known vitamins." They tested three grasses—barley, wheat, and oats—in the dried juice form. All were grown outdoors in the same field at the same time; subject to the same conditions, and all harvested after 30 days. According to Messieurs Kohler, Elvehjem, and Hart:

"The barley grass, which was the most effective, produced a growth rate of 5.3 gm. (weight) per day from the second to the seventh week of the experiment. The wheat grass was only slightly less potent than the barley grass....After 7 weeks on the experiment, the pigs....were taken off the supplement and fed mineralized milk alone. Growth stopped almost immediately. [Upon resumption] again remarkable growth resulted in the animals receiving the barley and wheat grasses. These results show definitely that the grasses contain a nutritional factor which is essential for maintenance as well as growth of guinea pigs."

The pigs receiving the oat grass did not do as well. However, the wheat and barley juice was so potent that it appeared to be all the animals needed to sustain life. This is surprising, because their digestive tracts are equipped to handle large amounts of roughage.

The animals receiving mineralized milk, orange juice and grass powder grew at a good rate and no abnormalities were observed. However, once the grass juice was omitted, the animals died.All the guinea pigs started out at 260 grams of weight. One group ate only lettuce, another only cabbage, a third only spinach, and the fourth only grass. On week 8 the cabbage pig was dying and grass was added to all the pigs' diets. All improved dramatically. Spinach was second best. The grass used was only 20% protein.

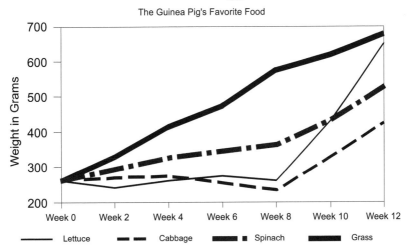

Grass vs. Veggies

The Guinea Pig's Favorite Food

All the guinea pigs started out at 260 grams of weight. One group ate only lettuce, another only cabbage, a third only spinach, and the fourth only grass. On week 8 the cabbage pig was dying and grass was added to all the pigs' diets. All improved dramatically. Spinach was second best. The grass used was only 20% protein.

Early Studies on
the "Grass Juice Factor"

1: Growth Stimulating Properties of Grass Juice. By G.O. Kohler, C.A. Elvehjem and E.B Hart. Science, 83:445. 1936. 2: The Relation of the Grass Factor to Guinea Pig Nutrition, by G.O. Kohler, C.A. Elvehjem, C.A. and E.B. Hart, Journal of Nutrition, 15:445. 1938. 3: M. Cannon, and G. Emerson, Journal of Nutrition, 18:155. 1939. 4: Distribution of The Grass Juice Factor in Plant and Animal Materials, by S.B. Randall, H. Sober, G.O. Kohler. Journal of Nutrition, 20:459, 1940. 5: Proceedings Cornell Nutrition Conference, M.L. Scott, p.73, 1951. and Poultry Science, 30:293.

In 1936, Kohler, Elvehjem and Hart reported that fresh grass juice contained an unknown factor necessary for the normal growth of rats. The rats were fed milk produced by cows that grazed on young spring pasture which was shown to be a good source of the water soluble "grass juice factor."[1] In 1938 using the guinea pig as his test animal, George Kohler found that the "grass juice factor" had an important influence on both normal and reproductive growth.[2] His findings were confirmed in 1939 by Cannon and Emerson,[3] and in 1940, the "grass juice factor" was also found in the young plants of white clover, peas, cabbage, turnip tops and spinach. The concentration of the factor was highest in the young grasses and reduced considerably as the grass matured. Other healthy foods such as liver meal and whey had none of the factor and brewers yeast and wheat germ showed only a little.[4] Experiments continued with turkeys and chickens, proving that these animals required the same unknown factor as guinea pigs and rats.[5] Baby chickens fed fresh grass juice produced a "marked growth-promoting effect."

Immune Function and
Growth Hormone Stimulation

Isolation of a Vitamin E Analog from a Green Barley Leaf Extract That Stimulates Release of Prolactin and Growth Hormone from Rat Anterior Pituitary Cells in Vitro. By M. Badamchian, B. Spangelo, Y. Bao, Y. Hagiwara, H. Hagiwara, H. Ueyama, A. Goldstein. Journal Nutrition & Biochemistry. Vol. 5: 145-150. 1994. Also, a-tocopherol Succinate but Not a-tocopherol or Other Vitamin E Analogs Stimulates Prolactin Release from Rat Anterior Pituitary Cells in Vitro. By same authors (except Bao). Journal Nutrition and Biochemistry. Vol. 6: 340-344. 1995.

White blood cells protect our bodies from infection and disease and are the front line defense of our immune system. The pituitary gland secretes hormones which control other endocrine glands and influences growth, metabolism and maturation. Barley grass leaf extract (BLE) was added to cultures of human white blood cells and to cultures of anterior (front) pituitary cells. The grass extract stimulated immune functions and the release of growth hormones and prolactin. These hormones are related to general health, reproductive health and other important physiological functions. This study successfully isolated and identified the molecule in barley grass responsible for this enhancement. It is a water soluble form of vitamin E called a-tocopherol succinate that is abundant in BLE. According to Dr. Allan Goldstein co-author of the study, "we now know that vitamin E plays an important metabolic role in maintaining the integrity of membranes and may reduce the risk of heart disease and lower the incidence of several types of cancer in humans, including breast and colon."

Other commercially available forms of vitamin E (alpha-tocopherol, a-tocopherol acetate and a-tocopherol nicotinate) were tested, but only a-tocopherol succinate stimulated the production of prolactin. This micro-nutrient suppressed human tumor cell growth in cultures where other tocopherols were ineffective. "This suggests a role of alpha-tocopherol succinate as an anti-tumor proliferative agent and as a modifier of human leukemia cell differentiation."

Immune System

Immune System Components Altered by a Food Supplement. Presented by E. Wagner and R. Mocharla, at the 1991 Annual Meeting of the American Association for the Advancement of Science, Feb. 16, 1991. Washington, D.C.

This double blind human study involved 32 first and second year medical students, 16 of whom received 6 grams of barley grass leaf extract (commercially sold as Green Magma) for 71 days. The other 16 received placebos. Everyone had a complete blood analysis before and after in which various components of the immune system were measured. The students who received the barley grass juice supplement exhibited a statistically significant increase in their leukocytes and a decrease in their lymphocytes. Their overall immunity was stronger than the placebo group. The authors commented that although no definite conclusions can be drawn, "one could hypothesize that the statistically significant increases in the percent of neutrophils and circulating complement levels, both components of nonspecific immune defense in the nutritionally supplemented group, could reflect a more efficient first line of defense."

Wheat Sprouts Increase Antioxidant Levels

1: Effects of Whole Live Foods on (SOD) Deficiency in 10 Adult Humans. Conducted by Dr. Peter Rothschild M.D. Ph.D. et al. Testing by Smith-Kline Bio-Science, Honolulu, HI. Antioxidant enzymes supplied by Biotec Food, HI. Courtesy of AgriGenic Food Corp. Huntington Beach, CA. 2: Calzuola I, Marsili V, Gianfranceschi GL. Synthesis of antioxidants in wheat sprouts. J Agric Food Chem. 2004 Aug 11;52(16):5201-6.

Ten senior citizens had their blood levels of superoxide dismutase (SOD) tested before and after taking a hydroponically grown wheat sprout supplement. The supplements were manufactured by AgriGenic Food Corp. *(see resources)* from the sprouts, a pre-grass stage of growth, using a low temperature process to preserve enzyme activity.

Young grasses are excellent sources of superoxide dismutase (SOD), a powerful antioxidant and anti-aging enzyme. This human study used 70 year old (average age) seniors who are naturally slower to respond than a younger population. Nevertheless, the serum levels of the seniors increased an average of 230 percent overall in the group and as much as 730 percent in one individual. Seven of the 10 participants more than doubled their blood levels of SOD. This proves that wheat sprouts are an excellent source of SOD and that potency can be maintained in a supplement. The high levels of assimilation are likely due to the fact that the supplement is a whole foods concentrate with all of its synergistic co-nutritional factors.

Wheat Sprouts as Anti-Mutagens

Mechanism of antimutagenicity of wheat sprout extracts. Peryt B, Szymczyk T, Lesca P. Mutat Res. 1992 Oct;269(2):201-15. Dept of Biochemistry, Medical Academy, Warsaw, Poland.

Benzo[a]pyrene (BP) is a highly carcinogenic combination of two hydrocarbons. In this study, wheatgrass extract reduced the formation of BP metabolites in rats. They found in the cell cytoplasm of the wheat sprouts at least two groups of heat-resistant compounds that showed antimutagenic activity. "The strong inhibition of BP mutagenicity with non-chlorophyllic wheat sprout extract suggests that chlorophyll is not the main compound responsible for the antimutagenic activity." They deduced that the antimutagenic compounds in wheat sprout extract must belong to its group of flavonoids.

Barley Grass – A Powerful Antioxidant

Inhibitory Effect of 2″-0-Glycosyl Isovitexin and a-Tocopherol on Genotoxic Glyoxal
Formation in a Lipid Peroxidation System. By T. Nishyama, Y. Hagiwara and
T. Shibamoto. Dept. of Environmental Toxicology, University of California, Davis.
Published by Food Chemical Toxicity, Vol. 32, No. 11, pp. 1047–1051, 1994. See
also the original study: A Novel Antioxidant Isolated from Young Green Barley
Leaves, Agricultural and Food Chemistry. Vo. 40, pp. 1135-1138. July, 1992.

This study tested fractions of young barley grass juice powder on highly toxic oxidizing chemicals to test the grass' ability as an antioxidant. Oxidation damage is associated with aging, cancer, HIV and other immunodeficiency diseases. Oxidizing agents reduce healthy compounds into toxic ones. When fats and oils (lipids) are oxidized, they degrade into rancid fats that react with amino acids and proteins and become hazardous to human health. This research examines glyoxal, a potent mutagen common in cigarette smoke. Living cells depend on enzymes and dietary antioxidants to protect themselves. Some famous antioxidants are vitamin C, beta-carotene and vitamin E (alpha-tocopherol), but there are many others in plants.

In this experiment, an antioxidant named 2″-0-Glycosyl Isovitexin (an isoflavonoid abbreviated 2″-0-GIV for short) was isolated from young green barley leaves. Its capacity to prevent the formation of glyoxal from degrading fats was measured. A kind of vitamin E, a-Tocopherol was also tested as a comparison. The amount of glyoxal formed from three different fats (fatty acids) in the presence of each antioxidant was measured. This was all done in vitro—in a test tube—not in an animal, and the results were replicated at least two times.

2″-0-GIV inhibited glyoxal formation by nearly 70 percent. "Alpha-tocopherol exhibited a greater inhibitory effect at the lower levels. On the other hand, 2″-0-GIV showed a higher effect than a-tocopherol at the higher levels. 2″-0-GIV is more effective than a-tocopherol towards fatty esters with higher numbers of double bonds. The more bonds possessed by a lipid, the more oxidation products it produces. A maximum inhibition of 82 percent was obtained by 2″-0-GIV." The antioxidant activity of isoflavonoids such as 2″-0-GIV was hypothesized because of their ability to chelate metal ions and scavenge free radicals. "In addition, flavonoid compounds reportedly affect many biological processes. They exhibit anti-hepatotoxicity, anti-inflammatory effects, anti-allergy effects and antiviral activity."

Anti-Ulcer

Anti-ulcer Activity of Fractions from Juice of Young Barley Leaves. By H. Ohtake, H. Yuasa, C. Komura, T. Miyauchi, Y. Hagiwara and K. Kubota. Issued from Pharmaceutical Society of Japan.

Until now, no evidence has been reported that pharmacologically demonstrates that grass juice can prevent peptic ulcers. This experiment created stomach ulcers in rats and then cured them with barley grass juice in 3–4 days. Rats were induced with different types of ulcers, treated with grass juice fractions, then cut open and the condition of the ulcers inspected. Seven different fractions of spray dried, green barley grass powder were tested along with a control.

Green barley juice revealed significant anti-ulcer activity in the various ulcers and one fraction "P4D1 significantly promoted the healing of the gastric ulcer induced by an injection of dilute ascetic acid into the gastric wall of the rats." On stress induced ulcers, all fractions of the barley grass exerted "significant anti-ulcer effects." The water soluble fraction GM-L exhibited the highest activity on stressed induced ulcers. Three fractions proved significant anti-ulcer agents against aspirin induced ulcers. None of the grass factors influenced aspirin absorption, gastric secretion of acid or pepsin. Therefore, the anti-ulcer action of grass is not a function of suppressed gastric secretion.

The fractions were composed of water soluble substances of chlorophyll, denatured protein, polysaccharides, amino acids, high molecular substances, and insoluble substances. "It is unlikely that green barley juice exerts its anti-ulcer action by affecting the attacking factors of the ulcer, but [it] suggests that the effects on the movement and blood flow in the stomach and the defense ability of the stomach mucosa are associated with its anti-ulcer activity."

Ulcerative Colitis

Wheat Grass Juice in the Treatment of Active Distal Ulcerative Colitis. A randomized double-blind placebo-controlled trial. Ben-Arye E, Goldin E, Wengrower D, Stamper A, Kohn R, Berry E. Scand J Gastroenterol 2002;37:444-449. Dept. of Family Medicine, The Bruce Rappaport Faculty of Medicine, Israel Institute of Technology, Haifa.

This full blown double-blind placebo-controlled trial followed a successful unpublished preliminary pilot study that also demonstrated the effectiveness of wheatgrass for patients with ulcerative colitis (UC). In this trial 23 patients with verified cases of bleeding colitis drank 100cc (3.4oz) of fresh wheatgrass juice (or a matching placebo) daily for one month. All patients were tested by four methods including physician exam and a sigmoidoscope evaluation. *Results:* Treatment with wheatgrass juice significantly reduced the overall disease activity, including the severity of rectal bleeding. In addition, using advanced cyclic voltammetry, they were able to trace prominent quantities of four groups of antioxidant compounds in the wheatgrass. *Conclusion:* "Wheat grass juice appeared effective and safe as a single or adjuvant treatment of active distal UC."

Antidote for Food Additives and Insecticides

Effect on the Several Food Additives, Agricultural Chemicals and a Carcinogen. By Y. Hagiwara, M.D. Presented to the 98th Annual Assembly of Pharmaceutical Society of Japan, April 5, 1978.

This paper presented the results of Dr. Hagiwara's tests on the ability of grass juice to inactivate mutagenic substances found in agricultural chemicals, fertilizers and food additives.

Barley juice extract successfully decomposed the agricultural insecticide Malathion, dropping its concentration down from 100 parts per million (ppm) to 19ppm in two hours. The food additive sorbic acid decomposed from 100 ppm down to 9ppm after 12 hours. The synthetic antioxidant and food preservative BHT was decreased from 400ppm to 40ppm after 5 hours of incubation with barley grass extract.

Detoxification of Common Pesticides

Degradation of organophosphorus pesticides in aqueous extracts of young green barley leaves (Hordeum vulgare L). Durham, J., Ogata, J., Nakajima, S., Hagiwara, Y., and Shibamoto, T. 1999, J. of the Science of Food and Agriculture Vol 79 (10) pp 1311–1314.

Detoxification is essential for any successful health restoration program. The overuse of pesticides in our air, water, and soil since the 1940s makes them so ubiquitous in our environment that even organic foods contain traces of them. That said, a method of neutralizing the effects of pesticides would be invaluable—barley grass to the rescue!

Drs. Shibamoto, Hagiwara, et. al. challenged some of our most vexing pesticides with young barley grass juice extract (BL) in vitro. They demonstrated that BL effectively degraded a range of organophosphorus pesticides such as malathion, chlorpyrifos, guthion, diazinon, methidathion, and parathion. When the above six pesticides were incubated in a 15% solution of young green barley grass juice for 3 hours, malathion and chlorpyrifos degraded 100%, whereas parathion degraded 75%, diazinon 54%, guthion 41% and methidathion 23%. They also confirmed that when BL is heated its ability to detoxify malathion is lost. *Conclusion:* Barley grass juice can help us detoxify our bodies from toxic pollutants in our diet and environment.

Pain Reduction for Heel Spurs

Efficacy of a wheatgrass topical application in the treatment of plantar fasciitis: an internet pilot study. Dr. C. L. Reynolds. M.B.,B.S. Melbourne, Australia
www.wheatgrassprofessional.info

Many people suffer from heel pain. Sometimes it is inflammation of the connective tissue at the bottom of the heel called plantar fasciitis (PF) or it can be a heel spur—a soft calcium formation. Since the heel bears the weight of the body and then some, patients can suffer for years and even walking up stairs can be excruciating. Conventional treatments involve surgery, steroid injections, anti-inflammatory drugs, shockwave treatment, and orthopedic shoes.

In this internet-based pilot study, PF sufferers were recruited from around the world on a first come, first serve basis. Thirty-one volunteers signed up, 13 males and 18 females, from the USA, Canada, and Ireland. Their ages ranged from 23 to 68 and had been suffering with the condition for as long as 12 years. Twenty had already tried either surgery, steroid injections or shockwave treatments. Participants were instructed to apply a "rice-grain size" of a wheatgrass cream and report their pain levels on a regular basis. None were informed about the known effects of wheatgrass. The study was managed by the semi-commercial website *HeelSpurs.com.*

By the end of the twelve weeks, four participants recovered completely, and more than half (16) reported a pain reduction of greater than 40 percent. Six experienced no improvement and one suffered increased pain and dropped out of the program.

Comments: This is the first time a wheatgrass product was tested for this condition. Given the anti-inflammatory effects of wheatgrass referred to elsewhere in this chapter, it should be no surprise that a wheatgrass-based topical product could provide benefit. Considering the results of this small, privately funded, subjective study, a larger, better controlled evaluation is warranted.

Stamina and Endurance

Studies on the Effects of Green Barley Juice on the Endurance and Motor Activity in Mice. By K. Kubota and N. Sunagane, Faculty of Pharmaceutical Sciences, Science Univ. Of Tokyo, Japan. Presented Before the 104th Annual Congress of Pharmaceutical Society of Japan, Sendai, 1984.

This study tested the motor activity and endurance rates of mice who had spray dried barley grass juice added to their standard diets. Thirty-two mice were tested, 16 with 2% grass added to their food and 16 without any as a control. The number of revolutions on their wheel cages was recorded over a two-hour test period each day for 15 days. The grass fed mice revolved the wheel cage more than the control mice in numbers that were "statistically significant." (Right chart)

On the endurance test, (left chart) 16 mice were prodded to race on an uphill sloped treadmill belt after 15 days of 2% and 4% barley grass added to their diet. "The momentum (body weight multiplied by duration) in the mice fed on 4% barley was significantly larger than that in the control group." "The average body weight of mice fed on the barley grass food was larger than the mice fed on the standard food."

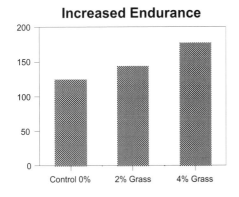

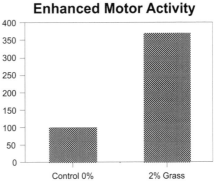

Dr. Ann Wigmore

"I separated six day old chicks into two groups of three chicks each. Each group was fed the best accepted type of chick food. But in one cage I mixed chopped up, freshly gathered wheatgrass with the food and placed a sprig of wheatgrass in the drinking water. At the end of a few weeks, all the chicks were healthy, but those receiving the wheatgrass had grown twice as large as the others. They were more alert and had feathered out better. Groups of rabbits and kittens, fed in similar fashion showed the same results in size, weight, and mentality."

Skin Diseases

Therapeutic Experiment of Young Green Barley Juice for the Treatment of Skin Diseases in the Main. By Tatsuo Muto, Muto Dermatologic Hospital. New Drugs and Clinical Application. Vol. 26, No. 5. May 10, 1977. Courtesy of Green Foods Corporation.

Treatment of skin diseases should include not only symptomatic therapy but also systemic therapy. In this long term clinical trial, 38 skin disease patients were selected for their resistance to conventional drugs. They had everything from acne to eczema to atopic dermatitis. A typical dose was 4 grams of green barley grass juice powder dissolved in water three times daily, either in between meals or 30 minutes before them. In addition to observations, blood, urea and liver function were tested. Considerable effects were noted in almost all cases in one to six months. "What was certain is that the administration promoted blood circulation, appetite, and bowel movement and the patients' complexions improved." One 43 year old male with gout and severe eczema on his back "had pain in his right leg and his uric acid was a high 8.6. After two months, it dropped to 6.5 and his eczema was completely cured." It even had an effect on leukoplakia, white spots in the mouth. "The ratio of effectiveness was 81.6% in all cases." There were no side effects. T. Muto concludes that overall, barley grass powder gives "excellent results cosmetically and in the prevention of aging."

The strong restorative power of green barley powder which is effective for preventing cancer, has the added advantage of making our skin beautiful. Dry, rough skin is associated with aging. —Yoshihide Hagiwara

Longevity

Wild-growing Edible Grasses in the Nourishment of Long Living Inhabitants of the Dagestan Republic. By Kh.I Mustafaev. Published in the Russian language periodical Voprosy Pitanieiia. Moskva: Biomedgiz. Vol.2, no.5. pp.27-31.Sept/Oct. 1993.

This study examined the diets of the inhabitants of the Dagestan Republic who are known for life spans of 120–130 years. The oldest recorded Dagestani lived to 146. The 2 million residents of this province live in the Caucasus mountains of southern Russia and east of Georgia on the coast of the Caspian Sea. Wheat is this country's chief crop and their diet consists of many wild grasses and weeds such as chickweed, shepherd's purse, rose hips, chamomile, lambs quarters, thistle, thyme, sorrel, yellow dock, vetch, daisy, clover, wild marjoram, oregano, amaranth, mustard, garlic, and the grasses of wheat, barley, and oats. They use the young leaves to make a raw salad and boil the older fibrous ones for soups and stews. Seeds are crushed and brewed into tea or ground into meal and used in breads and pancakes. They also make pickles and sauerkraut and, yes, yoghurt.

Researchers from the Caspian medical college examined 154 alpine residents living at altitudes of 6,400 feet above sea level and 24 living on the flat lands. Their families were also observed. The age of the test group was between 85 and 116 years old. Researchers lived with their subjects for 10–12 days, questioning them, weighing them and examining their diets and eating habits.

The "long-livers" wake between 5–6 a.m. and drink nothing but tea made from weeds and grasses until they take breakfast at 9–10 a.m., never before. They drink tea both before and after the meals for increasing appetite and improving digestion. The 90 year olds had the most raw greens in their diet of any age group but even the children ate greens. Researchers found the wild growing edible plants to be rich in B vitamins, citric acid rose hips, vitamin C and A and pectins. The plants contained other nutritional substances that were excellent natural stimulators of metabolism and digestion.

The flat-landers were not as healthy as the alpines but neither group had any signs of heart disease or hypertension. Researchers concluded that "many factors influence health including lifestyle, genes, heritage and work...[but] the location and altitude along with their unusual diet rich in young wild grasses produced their longevity."

Cellular Rejuvenation, DNA Repair, Anti-Aging

Preliminary Report on How Juice of Young Green Barley Plants Can Normalize and Rejuvenate Cells and Tissues, Repair Damaged DNA, Restore Cellular Activity and Prevent Aging of Tissues. By Y. Hagiwara, Y. Hotta, K. Kubota. Japan Pharmaceutical Development and Biology Dept. Univ. of CA, San Diego. Reported to Annual Japan Pharmacy Science Assoc. Meeting.

Damage to our genes (DNA) can be caused by many factors including everything from agricultural chemicals to medical drugs, radiation, x-rays, lack of enzymes and stress. According to Dr. K. Kubota of the Tokyo Pharmacy Science University: "A special fraction called 'P4D1' from green barley juice produced a remarkable stimulation to the repair of cellular DNA." Meiotic cells (the reproductive cells) are equipped with DNA repairing enzymes and binding proteins that can repair any damage to the DNA. Kubota isolated the meiotic cells and damaged them with x-ray irradiation and quinoline, both of which are carcinogenic. "When these cells were incubated under normal conditions, repair to the DNA was slow and some cells died. However, when P4D1 was added into the culture, the repair of DNA was promoted significantly both in time and quantity." No side effects were observed.

Activity of the meiotic cells decrease with age. However, "it is exciting to discover that this reduction in meiotic activity with age can be remarkably restored by the fraction P4D1. No stimulation of DNA repair or promotion of meiotic activity has been reported earlier from the use of any natural or synthetic product."

Inhibition of Carcinogens

Inhibition of In Vitro Metabolic Activation of Carcinogens by Wheat Sprout Extracts. By Chiu-Nan Lai, B. Dabney, C. Shaw, Dept. of Biology, Univ. of Texas System Cancer Center. M.D. Anderson Hospital and Tumor institute, Houston, TX. Nutrition and Cancer. Vol.1, no. 1. P.27-30. Fall, 1978.

This experiment took commercially available wheat berries and grew them hydroponically for 7–14 days into five inch tall wheat grass. Wheatgrass juice was extracted from the roots and leaves and tested against known carcinogens requiring metabolic activation. Extracts from carrots and parsley also exhibited inhibitory activities but not as potent as those of wheat. Unsprouted wheat berries soaked overnight did not demonstrate any inhibitory activities.

Prostate Tumor Cells and Barley Grass

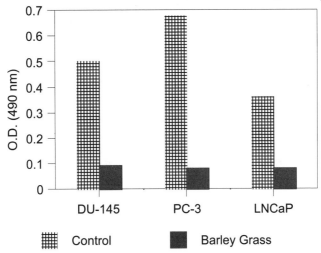

"These results are of interest for two reasons: first, the inhibition of activation of potent carcinogens is quite strong at a reasonably low level of extract and second, the wheat sprout extract is nontoxic even at high levels levels while most known inhibitors are toxic at medium to high levels." *(See also, "A Powerful Antioxidant.")*

Anti-Cancer

Anti-tumor properties of barley leaf extract (BLE) on human prostate, breast and melanoma cancer. Preliminary report by Dr. Mahnaz Badamchian, Associate. Professor, Dept. of Biochemistry & Molecular Biology, George Washington Univ. Medical center.

The above chart represents a preliminary report on the action of an unnamed molecule(s) isolated from barley grass leaf extract (BLE) that directly inhibits the growth of three human prostate cancer cells. The tall bars on the chart are the three cancer cells and the short bars show their reduction after BLE was introduced. Dr. Mahnaz Badamchian also found that BLE kills human breast (T47A, MCF7) and melanoma cancer cells. In all cancers, BLE proved effective both *in vitro* and *in vivo*. Human prostate and melanoma cancers were also grafted onto mice who then grew tumors which were "significantly reduced" with BLE. Work is still in progress on isolating and characterizing the molecule(s) from BLE that exhibit this unique anti-tumor activity. But should these preliminary results prevail, Badamchian states, this "could provide a novel nutritional approach to the treatment or prevention of cancer and present a potential breakthrough in cancer research." *See also: Immune function and alpha-tocopherol succinate.*

Anti-Inflammatory

Isolation of Potent Anti-Inflammatory Protein from Barley Leaves By K. Kubota, Y. Matsuoka, H. Seki, Faculty of Pharmaceutical Sciences, Science Univ. of Tokyo, Japan. Japanese Journal of Inflammation, Vol. 3, no. 4, 1983.

Superoxide dismutase (SOD) is well known for its potent anti-inflammatory action. Since SOD is abundant in barley grass, this study examined the juice of young barley grass and discovered that the anti-inflammatory effect was assisted by other proteins. These protein fractions were isolated and tested. Named P4D1 and D1G1, they are glycoproteins that are both heat-stable and highly soluble in water. In this experiment, male Wistar rats were induced with edema and then treated with the proteins orally, subcutaneously and by injection. No toxic signs were produced in the rats even at very high doses. Although SOD's effectiveness was significantly reduced with heat, "D1G1 was hardly reduced after heating to 100°C for 20 minutes."

"All of D1G1, P4D1 and SOD isolated from green barley juice revealed extremely potent anti-inflammatory activity, especially when they were injected intravenously. They significantly suppressed the carrageenan-induced edema in rats at very low doses..." Plus, both are chemically different from SOD and aspirin, also famous for its anti-inflammatory effects. "P4D1 and D1G1 seem to be much better anti-inflammatory agents than aspirin as far as they were concerned with intravenous administration."

Barley Grass Eliminates
Symptoms of Pancreatitis

Therapeutic Effect of Water Soluble Form of Chlorophyll-a and the Related
Substance the Young Barley Green Juice in the Treatment of Patients with Chronic
Pancreatitis by Osamu Yokono, M.d. First Dept. Of Medicine, Faculty of Medicine,
Univ. Of Tokyo. Courtesy Green Foods Corp.

Pancreatitis is a debilitating disease wherein the pancreas becomes inflamed, causing persistent abdominal pain, nausea, vomiting and high fever. The drug Trasylol is often recommended with mollifying results in the majority of cases but has side effects. While chlorophyll has been proven effective in treating pancreatitis in laboratory experiments and actual clinical trials, it needs to be administered intravenously which is neither convenient nor practical. Getting chlorophyll via foods is difficult because "less than 5% of ingested chlorophyll can be absorbed." The aim of this study was to discover the effect of ingested chlorophyll on these chronic symptoms. The food source was the freeze-dried extract of young green barley grass juice because it contains 1.5 grams of chlorophyll per 100 grams. Twenty-four chronic pancreatitis patients participated in this long term double-blind test.

"From the observations, we had the impression that the curative effect of the young green barley juice was obtained especially in the relief of abdominal pain. As for the so called side-effects of the drug, nothing unfavorable was observed clinically in the results before and after the administration of the drug, in urine analysis, hematologic surveys, liver function tests, kidney function tests and blood coagulation functions." But because barley grass juice contains "numerous known and unknown bio-active substances," these positive results may be skewed by substances other than chlorophyll. "Irrespective of the presence of uncertainty about the identification of the active substances contained in the young green barley juice, our results presented here suggest that the oral administration of the young green barley juice gives some definite favorable effects on the pathological phenomena related to chronic pancreatitis."

Lower Cholesterol for Type II Diabetics

1: Yu YM, Chang WC, Chang CZ, Hsieh CL, Tsai CM. Effect of Young Barley Leaf Extract and Antioxidative Vitamins on Ldl Oxidation and Free Radical Scavenging Activities in Type 2 Diabetes. Diabetes & Metabolism. 28(2): 107-114 (2002). 2: Yu YM and Tsai CE. Ldl Cholesterol and Oxidation Are Significantly Reduced in Type 2 Diabetic Patients Receiving a Barley Leaf Essence Supplemented Olive Oil Diet. Food Science and Agricultural Chemistry [published by The Chinese Institute of Food Science and Technology] Vol. 5 (1): 1-6 (2003).

People with Type II Diabetes are more prone to atherosclerosis. These two studies both from the nutrition and food science departments of two universities in Taiwan, set out to determine the effect of barley grass juice extract (BL) on lowering cholesterol counts for diabetics. The participants consumed 15 grams of barley grass juice extract in their diets every day for four weeks. *Results:* BL lowered total cholesterol and "act[ed] as a free radical scavenger" to slow down the oxidation of low density lipoproteins (LDL). "These results suggest that the production of oxygen-free radicals is effectively inhibited by BL." In addition, BL worked synergistically with the antioxidant vitamins C & E and with olive oil to further improve results. "Supplementation of BL in combination with antioxidative vitamins can reduce some major risk factors of atherosclerosis...[and] may protect type II diabetic patients from vascular diseases."

Prevention and Cure for Atherosclerosis

1: Inhibition of Malonaldehyde Formation from Lipids by an Isoflavonoid Isolated from Young Green Barley Leaves. By Y. Hagiwara, T. Shibamoto, T. Nishiyama, H. Hagiwara. Journal of American Oil Chemists Society, Vol. 70, no 8. Aug. 1993. 2: Studies on the Constituents of Green Juice from Young Barley Leaves Effect on Dietary Induced Hypercholesterolemia in Rats. By Y. Hagiwara, K. Kubota, S. Nonaka, H. Ohtake, Y. Sawada. Journal of the Pharmaceutical Society of Japan, Vol. 105, No. 11. 1985. 3: Inhibition of Malonaldehyde Formation by Antioxidants from 3 Polyunsaturated Fatty Acids. By J. Ogata, Y. Hagiwara, H. Hagiwara, T. Shibamoto. JAOCS. Vol. 73, no. 5. 1996

The peroxidation of skin lipids from exposure to UV light has been associated with skin aging and skin cancer. These highly reactive peroxides promote cancer, mutation and aging. The oxidation of fats (lipids) also plays an important role in the development of atherosclerosis, the buildup of cholesterol plaque on arterial walls. These studies show that antioxidants can counteract the oxidation of fatty acids and demonstrate results that are "not only preventative but curative."

In this study, freeze-dried young barley grass juice was extracted and broken down into fractions. The powerful antioxidant 2″-0-Glycosyl Isovitexin or 2″-0-GIV for short, was isolated from the grass juice. Its antioxidant activity was measured using gas chromatography analysis of malonaldehyde (MA), a relative of formaldehyde formed during oxidation of fats. 2″-0-GIV was compared with a form of vitamin E called alpha-tocopherol and BHT, a synthetic antioxidant used to preserve fats and oils in foods. Other comparisons included the high cholesterol drug Probutol. Several different kinds of fats were oxidized in test tubes of human plasma and replicated at least twice.

2″-0-GIV performed competitively with vitamin C, vitamin E (alpha-tocopherol) and BHT across the various fat oxidation experiments. While a-tocopherol scored higher in some tests, it broke down under UV-irradiation while 2″-0-GIV did not. "The antioxidant isolated from young barley leaves is more effective than the other two antioxidants (a-tocopherol and BHT) upon UV-irradiation." When vitamin C was added to 2″-0-GIV, it became more potent. The drug Probutol achieved slightly better results but by so little that it was declared to be just as effective. Just 2 units of 2″-0-GIV inhibited MA by almost 100 percent while BHT required 12 units and still failed to match 2″-0-GIV. "The isoflavonoid (2″-0-GIV) demonstrated significant anti-oxidative activity toward lipid peroxidation and furthermore can be obtained in large quantities from a natural source at low cost."

In the 1985 study published in the Journal of the Pharmaceutical Society of Japan, rats were fed high cholesterol diets and then fractions from barley grass juice extract. Their cholesterol was measured before, during and after. The grass juice fractions significantly lowered their serum cholesterol levels. "The present work suggests that green barley juice may be very useful for preventing humans from vascular diseases associated with hypercholesterolemia."

Blood Diseases

Wheat grass juice reduces transfusion requirement in patients with thalassemia major: a pilot study. Marawaha RK, Bansal D, Kaur S, Trehan A. Indian Pediatr. 2006 Jan;43(1):79-80. Division of Pediatric Hematology-Oncology, Department of Pediatrics, Advanced Pediatric Center, Postgraduate Institute of Medical Education and Research, Chandigarh 160 012, India.

Thalassemia or Cooley's Anemia is an inherited blood disorder where the patient cannot produce enough hemoglobin or they manufacture defective hemoglobin. Hemoglobin is the protein that carries oxygen around the circulatory system. Patients suffer from anemia, fatigue, shortness of breath, liver and spleen enlargement, heart failure, and other symptoms. The disorder mainly affects children in Southeast Asia (there are over 600,000 cases in Thailand alone), as well as those in India, Africa, and the Mediterranean. The standard treatment involves weekly blood transfusions or drugs with dangerous side effects.

The patients administered their own juice. They drank a mere 3.5 ounces (100ml) of fresh wheatgrass juice everyday. Many of them were children who didn't like the taste and could not keep up with the regimen. Nevertheless, even at this flawed level of consumption, the participants were able to maintain their hemoglobin levels with fewer transfusions and extended times between transfusions. Overall, 25 to 50 percent fewer transfusions were required. In his conclusion Dr. Marwaha stated: "wheatgrass juice has the potential to lower transfusion requirements in thalassemics."

Wheatgrass Induces Fetal Hemoglobin Better than Drugs

The thalassemia study above caught the attention of Professor Panos Ioannou a noted thalassemia researcher at the *Cell & Gene Therapy Research Group at the Murdoch Children's Research Institute, Royal Children's Hospital* in Melbourne, Australia. Professor Ioannou decided to examine the capacity of wheatgrass to induce fetal hemoglobin (HbF), a form of hemoglobin that is significantly higher in oxygen than adult hemoglobin. HbF can significantly increase blood oxygen levels for thalassemics and anemics. In fact, this is exactly the modus operandi of the intravenous drug treatments for thalassemia. In his in vitro experiment Prof. Ioannou concluded: "Our measurements suggest a 3–5 fold increase in the production of HbF by the wheatgrass extract. This is a substantial increase and could certainly provide an explanation why some thalassemia patients may derive significant benefit." Professor Ioannou's results with wheatgrass were striking and significant for three reasons. A) He used cutting-edge gene detection equipment that was able to specifically identify increased HbF production from the wheatgrass in three distinct red blood cell lines. B) The benefits were produced by a wheatgrass extract, the brainchild of Dr. Chris Reynolds of Melbourne. This shelf-stable wheatgrass extract worked in spite of the fact that it is virtually devoid of chlorophyll. C) According to Prof. Ioannou, the wheatgrass delivered new HbF at a level and speed that exceeded the existing drug therapies. In addition, wheatgrass is safer, easier to administer, and far less expensive making it more available to the underdeveloped countries where treatment is most needed.

Grass Juice or Whole Leaf

1: Proceedings Cornell Nutrition Conference, M.L. Scott, p.73, 1951. and Poultry Science, 30:293. 2: Unidentified Factors in Alfalfa and Grasses, by S.J. Slinger, Feedstuffs, p.8a. Jan. 21, 1956. 3: Anderson, G.W., Slinger, S.J. and Pepper, W.F. Unpublished results, Ontario Agricultural College. Guelph, Canada 1954. Reported in Feedstuffs, Jan 21, 1956. 4: Hansen, R.G., Scott, H.M., Larson, B.L., Nelson, T.S. and Krichevsky, P.J. Journal of Nutrition, 49:453. 1953.

M.L. Scott's research determined that the grass factor was rich in the juices of grass and alfalfa but was largely, though not entirely, destroyed by dehydration.[1] Dr. S.J. Slinger, commenting on the issue of whole leaf vs. fresh juice powder noted that "while the activity is partially destroyed by dehydration, there appears to be a significant amount of the factors present in certain dehydrated alfalfa and cereal grass meals. [But] juice preparations are more consistently potent sources of the activity than dehydrated products."[2] One study made a direct comparison of dehydrated whole cereal grass, sun-cured alfalfa and grass juice concentrate. They found that the grass juice, from a mixture of various field grasses and alfalfa, was superior to the whole dried cereal grass but not significantly so. Turkeys and other poultry grew equally well, indicating that the factor was present in the whole dried grass.[3] Dehydrated or sun-cured alfalfa gave a response at a dosage of 10% to 20% comparable to that of the grass juice at a dosage of 5%.[4]

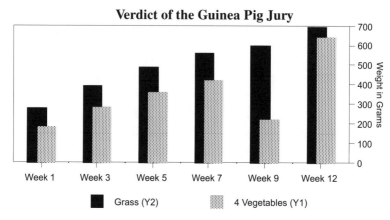

The Relation of the Grass Factor to Guinea Pig Nutrition. By G.O. Kohler, C.A. Elvehjem, E.B. Hart, Dept of Agriculture Chemistry, Univ. of Wisconsin. J of Nutrition, V.15, No.5. 11/24/1937.

Notice that even when four of our best vegetables (spinach, carrot, cabbage and lettuce) were fed to the guinea pigs, the growth was erratic and the pigs started to fail rapidly after the seventh week. To save their lives, dehydrated cereal grass was added to their diets (eleventh week) and in less than a week, the trend was reversed and a consistent and rapid growth took place. The experiments prove conclusively that while other foods are good, the grasses alone are the complete food and contain all the elements needed to support life.

—V.E. Irons *(see* The Pioneers*)*

Animals don't know anything about vitamins. They determine the nutritive value with their instinct, palate and olfactory faculties acting for them in place of judgement.

—George Sinclair, 1869.

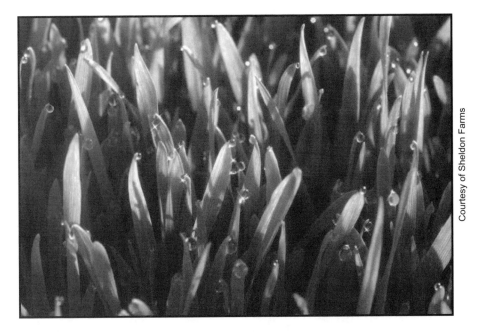

Healing with Grass
The Power Beneath our Feet

An analysis of blood samples drawn from more than two hundred Hippocrates guests before and after the two week program gave scientific support to our observations. Performed at the Arthur Testing Laboratory, the study showed that within two weeks of following the Hippocrates live food diet and drinking wheatgrass juice, the blood is detoxified and the immune system strengthened. These changes lead to more energy and an improved ability to combat and reverse illness.
—Dr. Ann Wigmore[1]

Healing is a Journey

Maybe you think that just by taking wheatgrass it will heal you. Well, you can drive from Florida to Alaska, but it's a long trip and your car had better be in good shape. Wheatgrass is just what your vehicle needs—oil for the engine, grease for the gears, fuel for the carburetor. You can't accomplish a trip like this without it. But when you finally roll into downtown Anchorage, it's the driver who gets the praise, not the oil.

However wonderful wheatgrass is, it is only the fuel energizer in your tank. Many people proclaim the virtues of wheatgrass and tell how it saved their lives. Wheatgrass gets a lot of credit. But it is not a magic potion. By itself, it does not cure anything. People do the healing, wheatgrass does the helping. You have the potential to restore balanced health as a result of the changes you make. Wheatgrass may inspire you to set out on this new path. But to achieve success, you will need to undertake a multi-faceted total health program. Such a regimen can take over your life. But what's your alternative? Sick people are often too stricken to function normally in society. These poor souls have to drop out either to die or to fight for their lives. So what if you decided to start drinking eight ounces of wheatgrass juice everyday. Would it save you? Perhaps. But it is still only the oil in your engine. By itself, it cannot spin the wheels. To assume that wheatgrass is a cure-all goes against the basic principles of how wheatgrass works. Call it the cornerstone of your total health restoration program.

The Causes of Disease

Health is a balancing act. Around 1980, world famous tightrope walker Philippe Petite walked from one tower of New York's World Trade Center to the other 1,400 feet in the air. He took his life in his hands for real. There was no parachute. Were he to make one false step, he would die. Everyday we take steps in our life that either keep us in perfect balance or throw us on a downward spiral. The fall into disease is not a single bad step, but a series of bad choices. Call them cigarettes, drugs, alcohol, junk food, poor hygiene, stress, work environment, air pollution, or water pollution—the result is cell pollution. The signs of disease are low energy, fatigue, poor digestion, gain or loss of weight, unclear thinking, allergies, headaches, joint pain and ultimately the major disorders—cancer, high blood pressure, heart disease, arthritis, emphysema, etc. Cells start to lose their life force. They misfire. Metabolism malfunctions. Organs weaken, digestion and elimination are disrupted. Toxins settle into the dead zones—the weak spots. Now the cells start to darken, choking on bacteria, yeast, fungus, and toxic acids. They can't get enough oxygen. Acidification, infestation, and destruction—the cycle of imbalance. We have fallen.

Rebuilding Health

The journey to rebuilding your health is akin to rebuilding your house. First of all, it needs a thorough cleaning. Forget about the mop.

Pull out the heavy duty vacuum, rent a floor sander, pull down the old wallpaper, rip out the broken cabinets, reset the squeeky door, spackle the hole, fix the windows. Although you may need assistance from professionals—the painter, carpenter, and electrician—you are the contractor. It's your house; you direct the nature of repairs; you choose the pace and you have to live in it during the renovation. Hopefully, you have not let things go so far downhill that you find structural damage. If you have termite infestation for example, that means you've ignored the signs and now you have to surgically replace a beam. If too many beams have been damaged, then the house may be beyond repair. There is a critical mass in any system beyond which it cannot recover. Although such deterioration does not occur overnight, it did happen right under your nose. You contributed to it by ignoring the signs and symptoms or taking wrong advice from the professionals. Or maybe you've just lived like a slob, wrecked the place and now look at the mess you're in. It's time to change your ways—renovate, rebuild, renew.

The Four Steps to Rebuilding Health
Cleanse. Nourish. Rejuvenate. Heal.

Step I. Cleanse

The path to health starts with a major cleaning. If there is infestation, you have to control it. If there is damage, you have to reconstruct. First stop the poisoning of the blood and tissues from acidifying diet, bacteria, yeast, giardia and parasites. Reverse the trend of acidification and alkalinize the blood with wheatgrass juice and an enzyme-rich living foods diet. Take nothing from a box or can. Eat from the garden. Eliminate sugar except when it comes from a fruit. Throw out the espresso machine and the microwave and put a juicer and blender in their place. Clear the blockages, empty the garbage, and reinvigorate the elimination system with colon hydrotherapy. Jump start the liver with a massage and a wheatgrass implant. You can change. Your body is a milky-way of trillions of cells that combine to make up tissues and glands. But every minute we breath in new atoms and exhale the old. In six weeks, every molecule in your liver is replaced. Renewal is a constant. What foods will you renew with? Stop treating your stomach like a compost and start treating it like a garden. Set in motion an upward cycle of rejuvenation that leads to balanced health. You'll begin to notice trimmer weight, clearer mind, brighter eyes, better concentration, more energy, and more vitality.

Many Diseases, One Cure

Although there are many diseases, all cures start with detoxification. Grasses, with their living chlorophyll, act in our bodies like detergents— purging the liver, scrubbing the intestinal tract, and oxygenating blood. Grass chelates and removes heavy metals from our bodies. While hemo- globin has a strong iron bond, chlorophyll has a weak magnesium bond *(see p. 48)*. Thus, wheatgrass readily releases its magnesium, creating a cellular vortex—a cyclone sucking in heavy metals. Tests on fecal matter, done before and after taking grass juice, show higher heavy metal counts after taking wheatgrass.[2]

Fasting gives your body a chance to re-balance its own chemistry, eliminating all the drugs and supplements that force it on detours and into different directions. Fasting is the great eraser, reducing all outside influences and creating a fresh start. Fasts of three to fifty days have achieved many miracles. Juice fasting with wheatgrass and raw vegetable juices introduces oxygen and nutrients into the bloodstream while en- hancing elimination.[3] From here, the reintroduction of 100 percent fresh foods gives you the potential for normalization and rejuvenation.

He who is immune is immortal.
—Lao-Tzu, ancient Chinese philosopher, founder of Taoism

A fully functioning elimination system is fundamental to any healing program. Colon hydrotherapy is a must. True, this is a much shunned topic that rarely succeeds as small-talk or acceptable party conversation. After all, it is the cesspool of the body. But herein lurks the origin of much disease. The colon is the exit door for putrefactive poisons. If the doorway is jammed, these poisons throw an extra burden back on the liver and start a cycle of auto-intoxication. Judging by the U.S. sales of laxatives, Americans have a lot of blocked doorways! Not to worry—one of the first noticeable symptoms of grass is its laxative effect.

The sweetness of tray-grown grass could be part of its power. Many believe the sugar helps to deliver grass' crude chlorophyll and phyto- chemicals into the bloodstream quickly. In the intestinal tract, sugars crystallize drawing out embedded toxins from the tissues. The powdered grasses cannot claim this feature because they have fewer simple sugars.

Profile of A Cancer Patient

In a study of new cancer patients at the Cancer Treatment Center of Tulsa, Oklahoma, most patients smoked or had smoked, did not like to eat green vegetables, had below normal body temperatures, rarely exercised to a sweat, ate large proportions of refined flour products (bread, crackers, cookies, rolls) had a stressful event in their recent history, and last but not least, drank soda pop, colas, coffee, bottled juices, and very little water.

The liver is the largest internal organ of the body and the most important organ of detoxification. It detoxifies drugs and removes toxins and waste products from the blood. A functioning liver is required for any health comeback. But too many chemicals from unnatural foods, drugs, poisons, bacteria and parasites can scar the liver (cirrhosis), or infect it (hepatitis) or otherwise overload it into dysfunction. Liver and kidney damage is the first step on the vicious downward spiral of degeneration. Wheatgrass has a purging effect on the liver and wheatgrass implants are the best way to cleanse and rejuvenate this vital organ.

The most striking thing was the appearance of their livers which were a dark mahogany color and the surface of the livers glistened like a mirror. The alfalfa-fed hens had light tan colored livers. These liver changes caused by good grass are too obvious not to have some connection with the prevention of degenerative disease. —Dr. Charles F. Schnabel.[4]

Step II. Nourish

Once the house is clean, it's time to rebuild. This is the fresh start you need. You are what you eat. If you are well, you can eat for entertainment and for pleasure of the pallette. But if you need to rebuild, you must eat for cellular health. An ill body is made up of trillions of cells, many of which are dying and malfunctioning. They need your help. Put away the pasta machine and get out the juicer. The best nourishment in the world is provided by enzyme-rich, organic, living foods. If supplements could do it, then our fast-paced society would have replaced lunch with a palm full of pills. Grasses, dried or fresh, are complete foods. Ask any of the grazing animals or the guinea pigs who nearly died on a diet of common vegetables *(see p. 60)*. It's not hard to find healthy living food. Just spend

Prescription for Healing

Cleanse

Wheatgrass
Pure Water
Detoxification
Fasting
Eliminate Parasites & Candida
Wheatgrass Implants
Colon Hydrotherapy

Rejuvenate

Wheatgrass
Massage, Skin Brushing
Homeopathy
Exercise: Yoga, Trampolining,
Swimming, Walking
Acupuncture, Chiropractic
Bio-Magnetics, Ozone

Nourish

Wheatgrass
Raw Juice Therapy
Living Foods Diet
Food Combining
Herbs

Heal

Rest, Sunbathing
Deep Breathing, Oxygen
Lifestyle Change
Spiritual, Religious Study
Personal Growth Work
Love

more time in the garden. (If you don't have one, start sprouting.) Many delicious and healthful foods never make it to the market. Eat sparingly and in proper combinations. As a society, Americans are gluttons, over-burdening our bodies with so much excess that it either turns into fat or ferments into a breeding ground for yeasts and parasites. Temperance is a virtue that will add years to your life and life to your years. Add grass, fresh or powdered, to carrot, celery, spinach, beet and other juice combinations. There are an infinite number of recipes available and you are certain to find a combination you love.[5] Explore the world of nutritional herbs and seek ones that apply to your condition.

It's not the food in your life. It's the life in your food.

Step III. Rejuvenate

Once the house is clean and the structure is strengthened, it is time to add the accouterments. Get the fireplace working, fix the furniture, re-place the appliances. You are out of danger now—the house won't collapse. But it is not fully ready to live in yet either. You dare not relax or else things could fall apart again. Although the pressure is off, you must continue your cleansing routine of grasses, colonics, enemas, implants, and a living foods diet. Expand your therapy to include regular massage. Start an exercise program appropriate to your condition—be it yoga, walking, swimming, or trampolining. Consult with other health professionals who can further your rejuvenation—chiropractors, homeopaths, acupuncturists. Explore different therapies such as oxygen therapies and bio-magnetics. Bathe, brush, and prune.

It's Easier to Stay Well Than to Get Well

Step IV. Heal

The ancient sages have long told us that healing is one part treatment and two parts nursing. And as any homeowner knows, it takes a long time to get things just right. Healing begs for creativity. When it comes right down to it, your lifestyle either contributes to healing or disease. Stress is the antithesis of rest. You can't change your health without changing your life. Attitude is healing; environment is healing; laughter is healing; love is healing. All the pieces of the puzzle have to be in place or it won't work. You are out of crisis. Now is the time for personal and spiritual reflection. Take classes in those things you have always wanted to do for your own growth. In this philosophy of healing, education is medicine; massage is medicine; yoga is medicine.

You can't change your health without changing your life.

Healing is not possible without rest. The fundamentals of health are very basic: oxygen, water, rest. It is amazing how long you can survive on just those three. When left to its own resources, an undamaged body will self-correct. Our lifestyle and our complex modern world get in the way, so for best results, retreat to a health spa. But if you can't make the time, then bring the "spa philosophy" into your home life: Take baths every day; Pour in some Epson salt or different herbs like mustard or ginger. Bathe in the sun. Brush your skin. Practice deep breathing exercises (pranayama yoga). You will be amazed at how powerful these simple practices are.

Your attitude is vitally important. For example, take the case of the first semester law students at the University of Kentucky. They were under tremendous, unrelenting stress. But of that group, those who were optimistic about doing well had more T-cells—the natural killer cells of the immune system—than they had before the semester began. The pessimists had no increase in their T-cells. These findings support the notion that thoughts and feelings influence the immune system.[6]

Wheatgrass—The Chlorophyll Cocktail that Cures

- Rebuilds the blood
- Increases hemoglobin production
- Heals wounds
- Cleanses the colon
- Anti-bacterial

- Alkalinizes the blood
- Neutralizes toxins
- Purges the liver
- Stimulates enzyme activity
- Chelates out heavy metals

Every disease is both strengthening and weakening. Many who have fought a major health battle are stronger for it. But years of living on the edge of illness is debilitating. Prevention of disease is one of the secrets to longevity. Our society is focused on achieving health through chemistry. If you have a headache, take an aspirin. If you have a stomachache take an antacid. If you have an infection, take an antibiotic. But these are not healers. They are symptom reducers. Healing does not come from drugs. If you want to achieve true healing—the restoration of balanced health from disease—include grass as part of a comprehensive wellness program.

Which Wheatgrass to Take?
Fresh? Frozen? Powdered? Indoor? Outdoor?

Everyone agrees that finding a convenient way to take your grass juice is the hardest part of the program. Powdered grasses are partly a response to that. What could be easier than spooning powder into a drink?

Wheatgrass differs from conventional therapies in that it requires more work on the part of the patient. The concepts upon which wheatgrass therapy is built are diametrically opposed to the pill popping style of modern medicine. Grass therapy involves the patient directly. Yes, it's hard work, but it is impossible to turn that responsibility over to your doctor or anyone else. Like Philippe Petite out alone on the tightrope, you are taking your life into your own hands. It takes courage and your life will never be the same. You will revamp your kitchen, your diet, your attitudes, your lifestyle, your beliefs. It will change you forever, but you will have your life back. You will have your health. You will have looked the Grim Reaper in the eye and said—Syanora Satan!

Dried vs. Fresh. Which is Better?

When Yoshihide Hagiwara developed barley grass juice powder, his goal was to make the benefits of grass juice as readily available to the masses as instant coffee. When Ann Wigmore started treating sick visitors at her Boston brownstone, she grew the grass in her kitchen and juiced it on the spot. After all, living in a big northern city apartment, what were her alternatives? Had she lived on a farm in Kansas, might she have grown it outdoors? She pioneered the use of grass to treat disease and her growing technique went hand in hand with her therapy. She squeezed the juice out with a grinder because that was all she had. Schnabel dried his outdoor-grown grass on his wood stovetop. Then he crunched it up and added it to the chicken feed. Subsequently, others have come along with different equipment and different techniques and have advanced. The whole process of growing and juicing grass is now more convenient and more available. After all, if there is a good idea, why shouldn't it evolve?

Grass is like fine wine. Different grasses offer differences in flavor, aroma, chlorophyll, and nutrition. Wine drinkers prefer some wines over others. But the general benefits of wine still apply. Wine is still wine; likewise grass is still grass.

All the evidence clearly shows that field grown grass is nutritionally superior to grass grown indoors in trays. And fresh foods are universally considered superior to dried foods. There are advantages and disadvantages to both. Science is not going to help you resolve this one (see *Science & Wheatgrass*). No experiment compares fresh grass and dried. But even if there was one, would you believe it? Would one study be enough? Surely, it would be disputed by the opposing camp. We live in a world where even the scientists cannot agree. In the end, you would still have to make up your own mind. So, here are the pros and cons to help you select the best grass regimen for you.

The original grass for human consumption was dried, bottled grass. This was the grass that healed the chickens *(see p. 60)* and was sold throughout North America in the late 1930s. All the university research done on grass, from then through now, has been on dried grass. These results are measurable and striking (see *Research*). No matter whether the grass is spray-dried, drum-dried, freeze-dried, whole leaf or juice powder, the nutritional value of dried grass far exceeds that of the fresh (see *Nutrition*). In the best processing methods, when you draw out the water,

Fresh Grass	Dried Grass
• Highest life force	• Concentrated grass essence
• High in sugars. 95% water	• Highest Nutrition
• Highest enzyme activity	• Some enzyme activity
• Labor intensive to juice & grow	• Very convenient
• Indoor grown	• Outdoor grown
• Tolerance: low dosage	• Tolerance: high dosage
• Patient compliance: low	• Patient compliance: high

you are left with a concentration of dry solids. (To learn about the different methods, see *Companies.*) These are the active ingredients— the solid content that contains all the plant compounds in preserved form. One thousand ounces of fresh juice can reduce to only fifty ounces of grass juice solids (this ratio varies). You can take large quantities of this grass juice concentrate easily and conveniently and you can have your choice of wheat, barley, Kamut, or alfalfa.

In contrast, the process of growing and juicing tray-grown wheatgrass could never be described as easy or convenient. Nor can you drink large quantities of it. Unfortunately, many people drop-out of the program because of the work load. Some have even hired nurse-gardeners to handle the growing and juicing chores. This raises the question: What good is a therapy that is too complicated to practice? If you can't integrate the treatment into your life, then it is just a nice idea. What's more, fresh juice drinkers need to drink ten to twenty ounces per day to achieve a therapeutic dose. Yet two to four ounces per session is all the average person can drink without upsetting the stomach. In order to treat disease, fresh juice patients must utilize enemas and implants. There are many plants in the botanical cornucopia with this same problem. The dosage required for therapeutic benefit exceeds the quantity consumable in the fresh state. Milk thistle, for example, is one of our best liver cleansers. Yet silymarin, its active ingredient, only comprises two percent of the plant. You'd have to eat a wheelbarrow of the stuff to get the therapeutic dose! On the other hand, milk thistle powder potentizes the silymarin content up to 80 percent. Now all you need is a gram of powder to start regenerating your liver. That's what dried grass juice is—a concentrate.

What good is a therapy that is too complicated to practice? If you can't integrate the treatment into your life, then it is just a nice idea.

Comparing Dosages

If you wanted to compare the dosage of fresh juice to powdered grass, you will find it is an inexact science. This is partly because one is volume and the other is dry weight. Nevertheless, here are some approximations to help give you an idea. Dried grass juice powder generally has a 20:1 ratio. This means that twenty ounces of fresh juice dries down to one ounce (dry weight) of wheatgrass or barley grass solids. This makes sense because fresh juice is 95 percent water. But wheatgrass juice powders are dried using different methods and their moisture levels vary between four and nine percent. Put another way, one heaping teaspoon of grass juice powder makes four to six ounces of rich green "reconstituted" juice.

Different Powders

Now you know that powdered grass is very concentrated and very convenient. But keep in mind that there are differences between powders. Some are spray-dried, some are freeze- dried, some are drum-dried, some are dried in carbon dioxide. (Read *The Companies* to learn more.) There are whole leaf powders and juice powders. Whole leaf means the leaves of grass were dried and powdered—including all the fiber. Some powders are ground so finely that they almost invisibly blend into the water when stirred. Juice powders, on the other hand, are made by juicing the leaves. The juice is dried until all that is left are solid particles—concentrated plant compounds that make up the essence of the grass. Because there is no fiber, this product dissolves easily in water. The juice product is more concentrated, but the whole leaf products are more economical and include fiber. Some people like the fiber because it is an important element in the diet. But it is non-nutritional. It offers no vitamins or minerals and slows down the digestion of the juice. Nevertheless, you will benefit from both of these kinds of products. You can read a study comparing juice and whole leaf in the *Research* chapter *(see p. 79)*.

But how do you know if you are getting a good quality powder? It all has to do with the method of extraction. For the moment, let's assume that all grasses are grown equal—Not! The factors that degrade nutrients are oxygen,

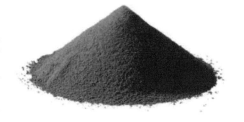

Spray-dried barley grass juice powder

Green Foods Corp.

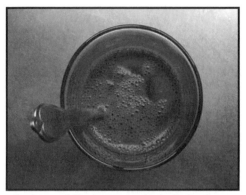

A glass of finely ground whole leaf wheat and barley grass from Nature's Greenz™ in New Zealand. With its rich green color it looks as if it was squeezed fresh.

heat, light, and water. The more a manufacturer minimizes the influence of these elements, the higher the quality of its product. How can you verify this? Here are a few things to look for: Enzyme presence is one of the indicators of high quality extraction. Super-oxide Dismutase (SOD) is one of those enzymes. It is abundant in grasses and also very fragile. If it is present, then the other enzymes are likely to have survived along with it. Chlorophyll is another marker. If temperatures are too high, it degrades into pheophorbide, a by-product metabolite of chlorophyll. High pheophorbide levels means there was some destruction of chlorophyll during the extraction process. Of course, chlorophyll development is also dependent on how well the plant was nourished and how much sun it was exposed to. What about vitamins and minerals? They are less fragile and they are also more abundant in the dried "concentrated" grass than in the fresh.

Indoor vs. Outdoor Grown—Which is Better

There are advantages to both indoor and outdoor grasses. So, no matter which choice you make, you can't lose. In the end, your decision may be based on some basic considerations such as taste, availability, cost, time, and convenience. When you grow indoors, you're in charge. You are the farmer and you control the product from seed to juice. You harvest it; you juice it; and you drink it immediately. You get all the therapeutic advantages of this fresh vegetable at its peak of enzyme activity.

Outdoor grown grass has advantages, too. Many love its mild flavor. Its long twelve to eighteen inch roots deliver an unbeatable constellation of organic minerals, vitamins, and enzymes. Its broad leaves provide a greater surface area for photosynthesis. Such exposure and slow growth turns the grass into a solar collector, storing high concentrations of energy in its leaves. That means one thing—more chlorophyll. This is, after all, the way grass has been growing for millions of years. Grass likes it

Outdoor Grown Grass	Indoor Grown Grass
• 60–200 days growth	• 9–14 days growth
• 12–18 inch roots	• 2–3 inch roots
• Cool growing temps	• Warm or regulated temperature
• Full spectrum Sun	• Lamps or filtered sunlight
• Natural breezes	• Fans circulate air
• Harvest before jointing	• Harvest before jointing
• Potential for E-coli	• Potential for mold
• Complex carbohydrates	• Rich in simple sugars
• Mild flavor	• Strong flavor
• Chlorophyll 0.4%–1.0%	• Chlorophyll 0.1%

cool. The cold temperatures cause it to grow slowly. Harvests come every sixty days and, if grown over winter, as much as 200 days. Indoors, the warm temperatures cause the plant to shoot up in ten to fourteen days. The indoor roots never have a chance to mature. Their two to three inch length is not quite ready to pull minerals out of the short two inches of soil. More minerals would mean more vitamins. However, because the indoor grass is such a juvenile plant, it is loaded with simple sugars. This is said to be one of the main reasons it has such a strong taste. The outdoor grass has converted those minerals into complex carbohydrates and has a more mild taste. Every indoor gardener has to contend with mold and insects. But mold cannot survive the wind and the ultraviolet light outdoors. That breeze has another advantage. Because the plant has to embolden itself against the wind, it develops more nutrients and protective compounds. More sun, more minerals, more vitamins, better taste... seems like a natural.

Can Dried Grass be Therapeutic?

Do you need the freshness factor or the intense sweetness of fast growing indoor grass to generate its therapeutic effects? Evidently not, if you read the research chapter in this book. There you will notice that most of the research was done with dried, outdoor-grown grass. Evidently not, if you talk to people using frozen, outdoor-grown grass, or read their stories in the *Real Stories by Real People* chapter. And evidently not, if you consider the origins of wheatgrass. It was outdoor-grown dried grass that Charles Schnabel used to revive the sick chickens in the 1930s. Even though outdoor grass is dried, it is still young grass harvested before the jointing stage. This is crucial to its therapeutic effectiveness. The plant is still in its prime even though its leaves are broader and its growing period is longer. Most of that growing period is spent developing mature roots, and that builds its superior nutrition.

Home Grown or Professionally Grown?

Should you grow the grass yourself? Or should you buy it from a professional? That depends on your time, space, and whether or not you have a green thumb. Most people would benefit from buying professionally grown grass—whether indoor or outdoor. There are some fabulous greenhouse (tray) growers out there. They know how to grow without mold. They know how to blend perfect soil. They know how to build the nutrition with super-fertilizers like seaweeds and rock dust. Some deliver to your door; some ship to your mailbox. (See *Resources*) Grass growers are dedicated folks regardless of whether they grow on thousands of acres or thousands of square feet. None of them do it to get rich. They are a devoted group who provide people with a quality product that when properly applied has the potential to restore health.

The Secret Power of Fresh Juice

You won't convince anyone that a re-constituted dried tomato looks or tastes as good as a fresh tomato. In any contest, fresh is always preferred over dried. But if you measured its elements, you would find that as tomatoes go, the dried is nutritionally well-endowed. So what is the missing link? What does the indoor-grown fresh grass have that the nutritionally superior outdoor-grown dried grass lacks?

When taking fresh-squeezed wheatgrass juice, people say: "I can feel it running through me." Or, "It makes the hair on the back of my neck stand up." The street kids call it a "buzz." They feel high. What is that? We call it energy— the life force. The Chinese call it "Chi" or "Tao." The yogis'—"kundalini." Yoda declares:

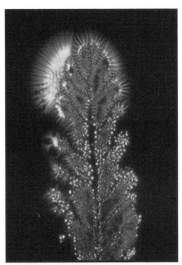

Courtesy of The Synergy Company™.

A blade of freshly harvested outdoor-grown grass. This "Kirlean" photo shows its electromagnetic energy field. This is the healing energy of living foods.

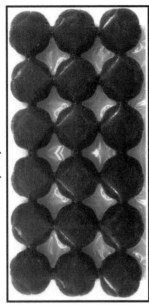

Courtesy of DynamicGreens

Convenient and potent.
Outdoor grown
wheatgrass juice
frozen into cubes.

"May the force be with you!" It is the electricity of vibrating, bubbling, scintillating life. Inside the juice, the photons, protons, electrons and quarks are dancing to the music of the cosmos. Our living cells reach out with an irresistible magnetism for these charged nutrients. This magical bonding occurs at an intensity only achievable between living cells. When we are ill and depleted, our cells operate at low intensity, like a weak battery. Only other living cells can provide the electricity we need to recharge. Although there is enzyme activity in dried grass, it is not at the same level of intensity as the fresh grass. There is a place for the dried product in your regimen. But when you really need to jump start a sick body, there is no substitute for fresh juice. If you are trying to heal and rejuvenate, you want the best. Juice the fresh grass and drink in the liquid sunshine. "It's the Real Thing."

It's powder. Anything that is dried has an incredible loss of vital life force. Even if you dry it carefully. Dried is dormant. Dormant is dormant. Problem with all that dried stuff is the life force–the ethereal energy is dissipated and lost. You're a living, vibrating entity. So when you drink something highly vibrational like grass—grass juice is the highest vibration—it tunes right into you and brings up your vibration. —Piter U. Caizer, the Wheatgrass Messiah

The best of both worlds would be to grow your grass outdoors and fresh squeeze the juice indoors. But that scenario is not possible for most people. However, some manufacturers do offer this in the frozen form (see *Companies*). You can buy it in the store or have it shipped to you by mail. These green ice cubes offer convenience plus the potency of outdoor grass. While frozen is not the same as fresh, it is pretty close. No, there aren't any scientific studies here either. But the testimonials of frozen grass users are just as impressive as any (see *Real People Real Stories*). And here's another idea. Why not hedge your bets and mix the outdoor powdered grass into a fresh squeezed vegetable juice? You'll get the superior nutrition of outdoor-grown and the "Chi" power of living juice. For example, organic celery, kale, and parsley are relatively easy to obtain—easier and more economical than finding a tray of grass. Now juice the veggies and add to it the best quality wheatgrass juice concentrate you can find. You've just made a formula that offers an alternative approach. It combines the best of both worlds. Bear in mind, the therapeutic dose for powders is much higher than the teaspoonful listed on the bottle. To treat disease, you need to drink ten to twenty ounces of fresh juice per day or the equivalent in powder *(see p. 91)*. While not a panacea, grass is a potent natural medicine in any of its forms: wheat, barley, Kamut, whole-leaf-dried, juice powder, or fresh squeezed.

How to Take Wheatgrass

Home Juicing

Home juicing is arguably the most economical approach to grass therapy. Volume users who juice four to twenty ounces daily for drinking, enemas, and implants, are really forced by the economics to grow and juice their own. But growing and juicing take time and effort. In Ann Wigmore's day, there was no other choice and many could not keep up with the regimen. Again, if your life is at stake, and your pocketbook is stretched, you will take the time to sow your seeds and clean the juicer. But today you also have other choices. Professional growers provide grass to health food stores in every major city around the world, and you can also have it delivered to your door overnight (see *Resources* chapter). Also, don't forget the wheatgrass retreats centers which offer multi-week programs where the grass is grown for you and the juicers are always running (see *Wheatgrass Retreats*). Many juice bars and health food stores also offer grass juice by the ounce. Today there is a greater variety of juicing machines available than ever before. For details on growing and juicing see chapters: *Growing It* and *The Juicers*.

Chewing

Just grab a handful and munch. This is the easiest way to get your grass and it tastes great, too. If you don't care for the taste of wheatgrass juice, then you'll love chewing it. Somehow the smaller quantities for chewing and the mixing with saliva mellows the sharp flavor of tray-grown juice. Since every mouthful is approximately ¼ ounce of juice, it can take about eight mouthfuls to get a two ounce serving. Beware: this could be a real jawbreaker! But, if you don't mind the oral exercise, whatever time you spend chewing, you will save in setting up, working your juicer, and cleaning the machine...and it's portable! If you pack a ziplock bag with two ounces of grass, you can take it anywhere. It's perfect for long drives and is functions both a breath freshener and an air freshener. Because grass is 95 percent water, when you finish it, you will have downed nearly two ounces of fresh juice.

The mouth is the ultimate juicing machine. While health aficionados debate the relative pros and cons of juicing machines (see *The Juicers*), all agree that the dentitious juicing apparatus preserves the most enzymes and offers the finest method of extraction. The biggest disadvantage is that this method limits you to nutritional and first aid dosages. You cannot chew the volume you need for disease treatment. Eight ounces daily is the minimum therapeutic dosage for serious illness. Two ounces per day is all that can be practically chewed. However, not having to deal with juicing, setup and cleanup time is the obvious advantage. One downside is cleaning up your teeth. Your new habit will be a boon to the toothpick industry! Grass finds its way in between everything. But you couldn't buy a better green flosser. Chlorophyll is a proven antiseptic and gum restorative. It tightens the gums around the teeth and successfully controls pyorrhea. But it is also like taking your jaw to the gym. It's a workout that will take some getting used to. That said, don't give up on your first try. It gets easier as you develop those jabber muscles.

Juice Bars

The next easiest way to get your grass juice is to drive to the nearest juice bar. Juice bars and smoothie bars that serve juices are popping up all over. Companies like *Jamba Juice* in the U.S., *Boost* in Australia, and *Crussh* in the U.K. are establishing hundreds of stores doing for juice what Starbucks has done for coffee. These stores know there is a juicing revolution. It's not hard to notice the one billion dollars worth of sales in home juicers. Also, health food stores often have juice bars inside. If they don't, they may sell fresh grass packaged for you to take home and juice. That saves you the effort of growing it yourself. In 2006, juice bars charged between $2.00 and $3.00 (U.S. dollars) for a one ounce serving of wheatgrass juice.

How to Make it Taste Better

If the intensely sweet taste of grass is difficult for you, try this. Grow the grass hydroponically *(see p. 172)*. It tastes milder and all the experts concur that this grass is still very potent. Also, try mixing it with other green vegetables. Celery is the best match. Its high sodium content nicely balances the sugars in young grass. Other favorites are parsley, alfalfa sprouts, spinach, kale, dandelion, and the sprouts of sunflower, buckwheat and pea shoots. Keep it all green. Add some garlic or ginger, too. You'll find it tastes like a liquid salad and the singular taste of grass is camouflaged. Finally, try growing your grass outdoors. This grass has longer roots, more minerals and a mild taste. It is completely lacking in the saccharine sweetness of young grass.

How Much to Drink?

Always drink any kind of grass juice on an empty stomach and then wait 30 to 45 minutes before drinking or eating anything else. For normal health maintenance, one to two ounces of fresh squeezed wheatgrass juice daily is typical. Therapeutic dosages are four to ten and some take up to twenty ounces daily. Although four ounces can be managed orally, higher amounts must be taken rectally. Wheatgrass has a strong cleansing effect on the digestive tract. It is close to being a green laxative. If you start off taking too much, you will find yourself running to la toilette. Nausea is also common with over-drinking and it is one of the reasons why therapeutic dosages are taken rectally. It's more than the chlorophyll that causes this because drinking bottled alfalfa chlorophyll does not cause diarrhea. Some say it could be mold *(see p. 165)*. Others say it is the enzymes and the intense flavor. Fresh wheatgrass is a high frequency enzyme elixir which jolts your system with a charge that is megavolts above anything else you eat. Even superfoods like blue-green algae can't match the "Chi" of fresh squeezed wheatgrass juice because it is not fresh. The secret to drinking wheatgrass juice happily is to gradually increase the amount as you become acclimated to it. Raise your dosage one ounce every three to seven days. Drink only what is comfortable. But if you are fighting an illness, you will have to take it rectally to achieve the daily ten to twenty ounce therapeutic quantity. Or use dried grass in quantity mixed with fresh green juices.

How to Take Wheatgrass Enemas & Implants

Ann Wigmore invented the use of wheatgrass implants. She realized that drinking large quantities can cause nausea. She also knew that only the higher quantities would provide therapeutic results. In addition, she believed that the large intestine was not designed to handle the Standard American Diet (SAD) of processed foods and fiberless flour products. Over a period of years, layers of paste build up on the colon walls, shrinking the tunnel diameter and reducing the efficiency of elimination. This is one of the causes of toxemia from which numerous aliments develop. Colonics and enemas assist in reducing the accumulation and restoring normal colon function. Ann started adding wheatgrass juice to the enemas which helped heal ulcers, sooth the tissues, oppose bad bacteria, and nourish the bloodstream. Since enema water is usually expelled immediately, she decided to first cleanse the colon with a wheatgrass enema. Coffee enemas were also used because of their ability to stimulate the liver. In a two-quart enema bag, only one ounce of wheatgrass juice was added. Once the colon was clear, from one or more enemas, a larger dose of wheat-grass was "implanted" and held for ten to thirty minutes or longer. Implants offer a way to introduce into your system ten to twenty ounces of grass juice. This is the therapeutic dosage required to purge the liver, purify the bloodstream, and detoxify the colon. These three effects are the primary benefits of wheatgrass. Anything that can improve the performance of the liver, cleanse and nourish the bloodstream and accelerate elimination must have a powerful, positive impact on health.

There are a few approaches to taking implants. For one, you could simply increase the dosage of grass in your enema bag. This approach is more wasteful of grass because much of it is flushed out and not retained. But the final round could have a higher dosage and is likely to be retained longer.

The standard approach to an implant uses a bulb syringe. First prepare the colon by cleansing it with a plain water or wheatgrass-water enema described above. It may take multiple enema bags to clear the intestine. A cleared colon is free of solid material in the waste stream and ideally, light in color. Now it is intermission time. Take a break to juice your wheatgrass so it is fresh for the implant. Pour it into a cup. Take a two to four ounce bulb syringe, available at drugstores, squeeze out all the air, then suck up all the wheatgrass juice in the cup. Grease the rectum with K-Y jelly or a water soluble lubricant. Either elevate your legs or lay on your left side. Squeeze the bulb slightly to eliminate any air bubbles; Insert and slowly squeeze. Rest for several minutes until you feel capable of taking more. Retention is more important than volume. Some people can hold their grass for hours. The longer the better. Small amounts may even be absorbed. Volume will be dependent on experience. Daily application and gradual increases are key. Although your first experience may be unappealing, you will develop the skills you need to enema and implant successfully. The benefits are worth the trouble.

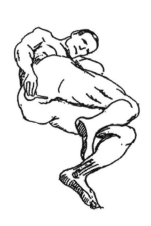

A few alternatives: If there is colonic hydrotherapy available, it is preferred. Colonics are more efficient than enemas and more thorough. They are also easier on the patient. You can accomplish more in one colonic than in several enemas. They're easier, faster, and more thorough. Another way to implant the wheatgrass is through an extension tube. This is a 12 to 16 inch enema catheter available by special order from your druggist or through the wheatgrass clinics listed in the *Wheatgrass Retreats* chapter. The catheters enable deeper delivery into the colon rather than just into the rectum. The catheter should be lubricated and inserted first. Then insert the tip of the syringe into the catheter end and squeeze.

Depending on your background, this may all sound very outrageous, terribly primitive or at least inelegant. But when you are fighting for your life, issues of dignity and grace go right out the window. This works, and in the end, it all comes down to choices. After all, chemotherapy is no picnic.

What If I'm Allergic to Wheat?

Many people ask: "If I have an allergy to wheat, can I still take wheatgrass?" People who have allergic responses to wheat and wheat products are usually reacting to gluten—the sticky protein found in the grains of wheat, barley, and rye. This is the same "glue" that is in plaster of Paris. The overconsumption of flour products in the American diet has overburdened our systems, forcing us to rebel with our allergic response. Its paste has also plugged up our intestines. Wheatgrass is different than wheat. One is a grain, the other a green vegetable. The green vegetable grass contains no gluten. It is no more "allergic" as a food than spinach, kale, chard or lettuce. In fact, it contains anti-allergic factors. Since allergies are immune responses to toxic irritants, detoxification is crucial to any allergy treatment program. As discussed, colon health is key. In addition to the liver purging, blood purifying and oxygenating capacity of grass, it coats the colon tissues with soothing, anti-bacteriostatic chlorophyll. Whole leaf wheatgrass powder also provides a high quality vegetable fiber—twice the fiber of bran—that maintains regularity. Add this powder to a daily juice to create a fiber-rich health drink.

Even if grass did have gluten in it—which it definitely does not—you could always switch to barley grass or Kamut. Barley grain has less gluten than wheat grain and Kamut grain has a different kind of gluten. The International Food Allergy Association found Kamut flour was okay "for most wheat sensitive people."

First Aid Applications

You do not have to be sick to use wheatgrass. Grass has numerous first aid applications from fatigue and sleeplessness to athlete's foot, bad breath, body odor and burns.

Eyes

When taken full strength and strained through a paper filter, wheatgrass juice has a variety of applications for the eyes, ears, nose and throat. Use

only one or two drops in the eyes for eye strain and tension. Slight sting-
ing is normal, but only momentary. Dr Gary Hall, medical director of the
Eye Surgery Institute in Phoenix, Arizona recommends wheatgrass juice
for anyone who shows signs of retinal disturbances or has a history of
macular degeneration. Because of its richness in magnesium, wheatgrass
acts as a smooth muscle relaxant which may be the reason glaucoma patients report relief.

Nose and Mouth

Placed in the nose, one or two filtered drops reduces inflamed nasal
passages and soothes mucous membranes irritated from allergies. Try it
for stuffy nose, sinusitis, rhinitis, bronchitis, itchy palate, etc. It easily
breaks through nasal congestion and doesn't have the boomerang effect
of drugs that leave you with even greater congestion after they wear off.
In 1941, Drs. Redpath and Davis, eye, ear, nose and throat specialists at
Temple University, treated over a thousand cases of allergy and upper
respiratory problems with chlorophyll and reported impressive results.[7]
Gargle with the unfiltered juice at the first sign of a cold or sore throat.
Wheatgrass' bacteriostatic and antiseptic action provide genuine relief.
It is also a great mouthwash and leaves your breath smelling fresh even after
eating garlic. Bleeding gums, trench mouth, gingivitis, and periodontal
(gum) problems in general are very responsive to wheatgrass.

*Based on comprehensive scientific evidence and my own
numerous clinical observations (over 25,000) since 1995,
wheatgrass and other cereal grasses appear to contain safe,
highly effective topical and systemic antigen-independent
immunomodulators. These confer on cereal grasses a
considerable number of important therapeutic properties that
sometimes, by their phenomenological nature, suggest so far
unrecognized physiological pathways potentially important
to medical treatment and research.*
—Dr. Chris Reynolds. M.B.,B.S. Melbourne, Australia

Cuts, Bruises, Rashes, Burns

Wheatgrass is great to have around the house for cuts, bruises, rashes,
burns, and sunburns. It speeds up the rate of healing and reduces scar
formation. Make a bandage from gauze dipped in wheatgrass juice. Even
better, re-dip some pulp back into the juice and put some of it under the
bandage. If it is a large wound, wrap it in soaked gauze or pulp and protect
it with a towel to prevent dripping. Repeat the process hourly for best results.

The American Journal of Surgery reported that in experiments with over 1,000 surgically wounded animals, chlorophyll increased the rate of healing by 25 percent over the non-chlorophyll control group.[8] Until you use it, it is hard to appreciate just how rapidly it reduces swellings, takes the sting out of burns and heals wounds—frequently without leaving scars. You can also use grass juice powder, either wheat, barley, or Kamut, for first aid. Just dip your moist gauze into the powder.

Skin and Cosmetic

And now for the cosmetics. What a great facial! Just dip some moist gauze into your favorite grass powder, rub it on and let it sit. You'll look green, but you'll feel great, and have a ready-made costume for Halloween! It's also a great skin cleanser, perfect for acne and black heads. There are documented results with skin problems like eczema (see *Research*), and it's been used for itchy skin, poison ivy, sores, boils, cuts, burns, insect bites and dandruff. Many skin conditions are related to liver and colon congestion and cellular hyperacidity, so in addition to topical application, you must drink the juice and get on a total health program for a long range solution.

Other Uses

Other reported uses of grass juice are: Hemorrhoids—make cotton-grass suppositories. Asthma and bronchitis—put compresses of wet pulp on the back and chest and drink the juice because it is an expectorant. Weight reduction—a grass juice cocktail before meals stays the appetite. Sleep—some users swear by a cocktail before bedtime. Eczema and psoriasis—Dr. Chris Reynolds, an Australian medical doctor has successfully treated thousands of cases using wheatgrass and his own wheatgrass extracts (see *Resources*).

Wheatgrass the New Miracle Drug?

Don't expect to find wheatgrass on your doctor's prescription pad. It costs 300 to 400 million dollars to evaluate a drug for FDA approval. Since grass is hard to patent, drug companies are not likely to make that investment. The basic approach of modern medicine is to treat physical abnormalities with chemistry and surgery. Wheatgrass does not fit into this model. Fresh wheatgrass juice enlivens the spiritual in addition to nourishing the physical. It's an electrical elixir transmitting a charge of energy that arcs across neurons and nerve fibers, revitalizing trillions of cells. From the conventional medical standpoint, it's quackery. Nonetheless, the medical establishment has been forced to expand their perspective before—on therapies as mysterious as acupuncture. No, wheatgrass is not a magic potion. But when used as part of a total health revitalization program with an indefatigable commitment to wellness, it is a powerful botanical medicine that enhances and maximizes your full healing potential. (For more, see *Science & Wheatgrass*.)

The cure of many diseases is unknown to the physicians... because they are ignorant of the whole, which ought to be studied also; for the part can never be well unless the whole is well... [This] is the great error of our day in the treatment of the human body, that the physicians separate the soul from the body. —Plato, 477–347 BC.

Real Stories from Real People

With my fitness level, my drive and desire, I'm not going to lose. I can't lose. —Lance Armstrong, USA Cycling champion on his battle against testicular cancer

The stories in this chapter are the testimonies of real people in their own words. These are people whose lives have been threatened, often by a terminal illness. Many have been sent home to write their will or told they only had a short time to live. They are not "health nuts" or "extremists." Many have never even heard of wheatgrass before. They are plain folks for whom conventional medicine has done all it can. But they had the will to live and therefore sought out and embraced alternative treatments. Their lives cannot be dismissed as anecdotal evidence. These are real lives, real struggles, and real personal crises. Some cases involve animals—beloved pets whose owners desperately fought to save them. Animals provide another level of evidence because they do not experience "faith healing," or a placebo effect. The stories herein represent only a fraction of the hundreds and thousands out there. They are not provided as "proof." They are presented as hope. Comments, questions, and/or clarifications inside the brackets [ ] are the author's.

Brain Tumor

—Pastor Lindsey Robinson, Harrisburg, PA
Wife Myra Robinson's comments are presented in italics.

It was the Monday after Thanksgiving 1999, I got up that morning, I was feeling so weak I could hardly get myself together. A friend of mine at work offered to drive me to the hospital. After a week in the hospital, they couldn't figure out what was wrong with me even though they gave me every test they could think of. I went back at the end of January and the doctor told me I had a brain tumor. *[Myra Robinson:] It was glioblastoma multiforme, (GBM), the most common, and most aggressive of the primary brain tumors, in addition to being the most resistant to treatment.*

He said he couldn't touch it because it was near some nerves and if he touched it in any way, I could be paralyzed on my right side. I wanted another opinion so I went to Johns Hopkins Hospital in Baltimore. They said they could take some of it out. So, they did operate in April 2000.

After the operation, I was just going about my duties and all. I'm a pastor, so I prayed. I went back for an MRI and so forth, twice per year and I thought everything was okay. But in 2004, one MRI showed renewed activity. *The scan showed significant activity. This time the tumor was stage four. Stage five is the highest.* When I heard that I got really concerned and went in for a second surgery in Feb. 2004 by the same doctor, Dr. Raphael Tamego at Johns Hopkins. He told me that I only had a short time to live, but they also wanted to give me the benefit of the doubt. So, while I was recuperating, they gave me thirty three consecutive radiation treatments. And it didn't do me any good at all. All it did was mess up my right side. Now I have to walk with a cane in my left hand because my right side and my right leg are all messed up. The treatments just sapped all the strength out of my right side. I couldn't hold my arm up very long, and I had to sit down a lot.

Thirty three treatments was the maximum allowed. He also had one week of chemotherapy. By the end of May, my husband appeared to have had a stroke. His entire right side was useless—his right foot dragged, he was unable to use his right hand, and his speech was slurred. An MRI showed that, in spite of the radiation and chemotherapy, the tumor had not responded to treatment at all and was in fact, more aggressive than ever. The radiation had caused the brain to swell resulting in his physical debility. He was treated with high doses of steroids administered intravenously to reduce the swelling.

So I woke up one day and I was just so weak again. So my wife took me to Hershey Medical Center. My family heard how sick I was so they all came here to see me. But the doctors said there was nothing else they could do. *We were given information about Hospice care and sent home, where he was bedridden for a month.* My cousin from Chicago mentioned to my wife, "Have you heard about wheatgrass juice?" She said no, she had not. So they got on the computer and found this man up in Canada who sells it. So my cousin paid for the first shipment. It comes frozen. My wife makes it up for me each day and I drink about six ounces at a time. Now, I'm not going to say that this is the cause, because I cannot tell you for sure, but I can remember the tumor shrinking during the time after I started taking the wheatgrass juice. The last three MRIs that I had, each one shows it shrinking and I'm praying now for it to be eradicated.

Although he uses a cane, his walking has greatly improved; he has regained the use of his right hand, has experienced general strengthening on the right side of his body. He is able to stand for longer periods of time, is able to drive around the city for short trips, and although he has to sit, has returned to preaching.

Now, here's the funny part, when I was in the hospital last time, my doctor came in and told me there was no hope for me. My wife asked how long does he have, and they said he'll be gone by the summer. *He said, "We have done all that is medically possible."* Well, that's over one year ago and I'm still here. The oncologist said "The tumor is shrinking, but I don't know why." So he put me on the oral chemotherapy drug Temador, a low dose. I take it for five days, every 23 days. *We continue to give God all glory and praise, for He has indeed done a wonderful thing!*

Breast Cancer, Skin Problems

—Tom Stem, Dog Breeder. Shetland Sheep Dog and Irish Wolfhound. Stouffville, Ontario, Canada

I am a longtime breeder of Shelties (Shetland Sheepdogs) and Irish Wolfhounds. Since 1969, I have kept twenty to twenty-five adult dogs in my kennel. In case you don't know it, cancer is the major cause of death for the Irish Wolfhound. But for both these breeds, when they get sick, it is either cancer or liver problems, or problems with the kidneys, skin, or bones. All their illnesses fall under these categories. By being proactive with sound nutrition and the use of wheatgrass juice our dogs have been able to avoid most of these ailments.

Breast Cancer

We got started feeding the dogs wheatgrass because of my wife. Janice was diagnosed with breast cancer in 1972. In fact, the doctor booked her for surgery within a week of the office visit. She had a grayish appearance and a deep seated level of fatigue. We accepted the accuracy of the diagnosis, but we immediately started looking at alternative therapies. We got the book "How I Conquered Cancer Naturally" by Eydie Mae Hunsberger and were inspired by the Ann Wigmore program. We decided to cancel the surgery and try wheatgrass juice therapy. We grew the wheatgrass ourselves and Janice drank about eight ounces per day, every day. After about nine months of continuous wheatgrass juice, the lumps in the breast disappeared. The oncologist gave her a clean bill of health. He didn't ask any questions and he even forgot that she had cancelled the surgery!

But there's more to the story. We had lots of leftover pulp from the juice we were using for Janice. So I started putting some of it in the feed bowls for the dogs. It still had a little juice in it. I mixed it in with meat, vegetables, and a little water. Later, after I started growing the grass outdoors (and freezing the juice to preserve it), I would just add a few cubes to the bowl and they would chew on it like candy.

Fertility

Neither of these breeds can mother puppies after six to seven years of age and most breeders consider this a limitation of their natural fertility. But my dogs have had litters as old as ten years. And the size of the litter for the Shelties is generally two to four puppies. But my Shelties have litters of five to seven puppies! Even if I was not a believer, as a business man, I would include wheatgrass in the diet because it makes money. Each puppy sells for $600–$700, and I get two more puppies per litter than the average breeder!

Longevity

Typically a Sheltie that is fed purely commercial food, lives only seven or eight years. If their diet is a mix of commercial food and owners throwaway food from the table, they can live for ten to eleven. Our Shelties generally live from fourteen to seventeen years. In the case of the Irish Wolfhound, they only last four to five years when fed a commercial dog food diet. When they are fed a mix of commercial food and scraps from the owners table, they live six to seven years. Most of ours make it to nine years old.

No one will face the brutality of this truth. It is highly controversial because few will acknowledge the role of diet in aging and health. They just consider it a genetic weakness. But I've seen what quality nutrition will do and I know what commercial dog food will do. I've seen puppies who need to be put down because they never developed strong enough bones in their legs. The back legs grow crooked. Their skeletons are weak from malnutrition. It's akin to rickets in humans.

Skin Problems

Some people started to bring me their sick dogs. I find that skin problems respond very quickly to wheatgrass juice. I can even tell you one case where the skin was actually weeping, it was so irritated. The doctors put her [dog] on steroids to try to control it. At first the drug worked, and then it just didn't work anymore. They were going to put the dog down when they brought her to me. At that point, I decided to try one ounce of wheatgrass juice per twenty lbs. of body weight per day. Well, in seven days, you could see improvement in the open sores. After two weeks, there was a little fuzz of hair starting to grow back over the bald spots. After three weeks, the hair was starting to cover the old sores. Her disposition was normal and she was looking healthy. When the owner came back, she got such a joyous reception she said, "My dog is acting like a puppy again!"

Veterinarian

What does the vet have to say? Throughout this entire time, we have used the same veterinarian, Dr. Clark of Sharon Veterinarian Clinic. It was Dr. Clark who actually triggered our focus on all this by asking me, "Why don't I ever see one of your dogs with cancer?" "Do you see much cancer?" I asked. "Oh, I see it every week, but never from you!" So I started to think, what is it? Is it that we use large outdoor runs? I don't think so. And the only thing was the wheatgrass juice. In the time since I started adding the wheatgrass, we have never had a dog with cancer, never had any liver troubles, nor kidney, skin, or skeletal problems. I am absolutely convinced it is the wheatgrass.

Confirmation

This was in the early days of using the wheatgrass juice and I still wanted confirmation. So I asked Dr. Clark to send me a dog with cancer. It happened that someone had brought her a very old Irish Wolfhound that was going to be put down. She was in considerable pain. She had a tumor on her front leg and couldn't use it at all. She couldn't even touch the floor with it. The owner gave me the dog to try to do what I could. So I made her a comfortable bed and fed her four to five ounces of wheatgrass per day. I really didn't know what I was doing then. Today I would feed eight to ten (ounces). I really wanted to make sure she got it so I fed her through a syringe down her throat. In a matter of a few days, the dog was obviously more comfortable. After a week she was tentatively reaching out with that foot. After two weeks, she was lightly touching the floor with it. After a month, she was walking. She never did run again. The tumor was still there, and it was large and hard as a rock. But she got full mobility and use of that joint. She was able to trot and was clearly enjoying life, socializing with the other dogs.

About four months later, when Dr. Clark was here for other work, she saw the dog. And I can tell you her reaction was one of absolute astonishment—total disbelief that the dog was still alive. The dog went on to live for nine months, which is a long time for an elderly Irish Wolfhound with terminal cancer. I would have given her more juice had I known what I know now. But still I was completely able to return the dog to normal activity. I want you to know, I am not embellishing this story or anything else I've been telling you. This is absolutely what happened and what I observed.

Colon Cancer
—Michael Claener, Queensville, Ontario, Canada

I went to my doctor for a normal check up and blood test and he informed me that my blood count was low. He was concerned and wanted to check it again. Before I go on, I should tell you that my immediate family and my relatives are all in dentistry or medicine. While that doesn't make me a professional, I was brought up in an environment in which I had a very solid understanding what these fields were all about.

When I left my doctor's office I knew there was a problem, but I tried to convince myself that in thirty days the test results would be normal and that would be the end of it. Well, over the course of the next thirty days I watched my stools closely and they were getting darker. I knew within my heart of hearts that I had a problem. I returned to the doctor, but told him nothing about what I saw. On this next test, the blood count had dropped again. I was losing blood. He started to discuss taking further action but I stopped him. I just refused to do anything invasive. I told him I wanted to do the test again. There was definitely blood in the stool and it was very scary. On the next test, my count had dropped to twenty-one.

That was alarming because it should have been a minimum of thirty four and it kept getting lower. He asked me to do a stool test and I told him it didn't need to be done. It was black [from blood]. He said, "I know your family and I also know that you understand the problem (colon cancer). We need to get at it sooner rather than later." I told him I would get back to him and quickly left his office.

So then, for the first time, I called my cousin who is an oncologist. He said, "Michael, it's only one thing. With blood in the stool and the blood count so low, there is no question. It's colon cancer. That's what you've got." He told me to have a colonoscopy and have it removed. My brother is also a doctor and I got the same lecture from him. But I refused to do anything invasive. I wouldn't let them touch me. I know these guys, oh, we're gonna fix it, and then they go in there and start cutting and probing, and then before you know it, the cancer is spreading, and then you're on your death bed. So I made my mind up–I'm not going there!

My decision was to try wheatgrass. I felt that I had nothing to lose. I went on a crash program taking eighteen ounces of wheatgrass juice every day (frozen wheatgrass, outdoor grown). I never did the colonoscopy and I didn't go back to the doctor for three months. Why should I? I knew what he was going to say and I didn't want to hear it. But my head was definitely in the right place because I could see my stool color getting lighter. After three months on wheatgrass, I took another test and my blood count was back up to thirty three. That's almost normal. My doctor couldn't believe the results. He said: "Maybe you're just having a good day. Let's test it again to be sure." On the next month's test, my blood count went up to thirty eight, and the one after that, it went to thirty nine. The doctor...he just scratched his head. I wouldn't tell him it was wheatgrass because I didn't want to get into a whole debate.

That was at age fifty six. I'm fifty nine now and I have never looked back. It was a really scary time for me. In my view, anybody facing such news, and who, like me, does not want to do anything surgical, has nothing to lose by trying wheatgrass. I will also tell you that the will to win must be there as well. I know throughout that time, my attitude was...I was going to lick this killer.

Heart, Stomach, and Throat Cancer

—*Edward Brown, MD. Los Angeles, California*

I graduated medical school in '72 and immediately joined a local clinic that was dedicated to working with the poor. We provided medical treatment to people who could not afford it. It has not been a money making career, but the work has been good to me. I've gotten to see the world—the Carribean, Central America, the Philippines, Australia...I call myself a jungle doctor. It's missionary work. I don't have a license in the U.S. anymore.

I discovered I had cancer in 1989. It was a rare terminal cancer, a growth inside my heart. I had four heart attacks. Each time it got worse. The lump got bigger and it started spreading. I had to stop working, although I did some volunteer work to keep my mind off my troubles.

Cancer took my life on a new journey. Because I had it, I specialize in it now. It has become my life's work. When I began to research my options, I was disappointed that there weren't any good solutions out there–only slicing, chemo, and radiation.

Well, that took me from 1989 to 1994. I had my last heart attack in '94. The tumor had finally pulled away. But it was entwined inside the nervous system that feeds the heart. The heart was sharing blood and nerves with the tumor. So, there were many small "disruptions." But my tumor eventually dissolved, and that's with verification. What saved me, without a doubt, was juice therapy. Unfortunately, I was not aware of wheatgrass at that time. I wish I was. But in the last six months of my healing, I juiced 80% of what I ate. I was on a mostly raw, vegan diet, with some brown rice. Before I started juicing, the tumor was stable, but it wasn't shrinking. Another MD told me that lack of cellular hydration [not enough fluids in the cells], creates a breeding ground for the spread of the cancer. So, I thought, the best water, water that is healthy and alive, is the kind inside fruits and vegetables. Juice therapy is the best therapy I know. And wheatgrass is the best vegetable you can juice. Eighty percent of what you eat should be drunk. Juicing, and good diet will replenish, nourish, and rehydrate you at the cellular level.

That's one of the reasons I like wheatgrass. Because pound for pound, dollar for dollar, I find wheatgrass is the most effective way to prevent and treat a variety of conditions. Terminal patients get to a certain stage where they cannot eat anymore, but you can always get wheatgrass into you. If you can't drink it, you can get it through an enema. You can soak your body [bathe] in it. Through any of these ways, it will get into your capillaries. If I had only one product to give to a patient, it would be wheatgrass. Even for years, if that's all you had [for sustenance], you would never die of starvation. I've been to so many countries, and used many wonderful [natural] medicines. But unfortunately, they only work for some people. Wheatgrass works for everybody. I've seen it over and over again. That's been my own experience.

If I had only one product to give to a patient it would be wheatgrass. —Edward Brown, MD

Wheatgrass does phenomenal things for cellular regeneration. Yes, there are other phenomenal technologies out there. But I don't care what you've got, if you don't have a strong foundation of nutrients in the blood, they're not going to work...or only temporarily. The first thing I do with people is get them started on wheatgrass.

Pain Management

I have clients right here in Canada, [for whom] the other doctors say [to them], "Look, how can you tolerate the pain? You should be on morphine!" And they ask me, "What are you doing to eliminate pain?" I say, "Well, I do a lot, but if I were to point to one thing, it would be the wheatgrass." It is a major anti-inflammatory. It's just the best one, but you have to use high doses. Ten to fifteen ounces per day. Feed a little each hour from 10am-8pm. Slow intake every hour.

[Are you committed to outdoor grown grass?] I guess so. With the tray grown, you ultimately run the risk of allergy, especially because some people don't grow it well and it gets moldly. Some people are allergic to that. And also, many people find the taste objectionable. When I see them after a while, I find out they've quit. I say, "Why?" And it's because they couldn't bear the taste. The outdoor never has mold. We just don't see the allergies there and it tastes great. *[How much of it is frozen grass?]* Most of it. All of it, really. It's the only way you can get it [outdoor grown]. And it's easier than growing it yourself. But whatever [wheatgrass] you choose, it's fine with me.

Throat Cancer

Now here is a phenomenal case. I went to see a little ten year old girl. She was diagnosed with Rhabdomyosarcoma. It is a fast-growing, highly malignant tumor. This is the most common soft tissue sarcoma in children. It's actually a kind of primitive muscle cell that grows out of control and it is most often in the head and throat. And they're big. This one was so massive that it actually grew out of her mouth. It was the size of man's fist. She had two years of chemo and radiation and then they sent her home to die. She was not able to eat anything. Anything you put into her mouth, she threw up. I came on board and introduced wheatgrass. I fed it through a feeding tube. First time, she threw it up. But after that, she was able to take it. And it absolutely turned her around. It took a long time. But the tumor got smaller and smaller. Eventually, this kid was going out everyday, driving on her father's golf cart and riding her horse. If it weren't for the wheatgrass, she would not have made it. You probably don't want to write about this one because it wasn't a happy ending. She died. But not from her cancer. Her tumor was gone and out of her mouth. We have the pictures before and after. She survived her cancer. But she choked to death, and that is another story–one that absolutely infuriates me. It was a medical decision not to do a surgical procedure to help her breathe better. That has to do with the politics of the medical world up here [Canada].

Stomach Cancer

I currently have a patient with stage 5 cancer, and that usually means they will survive only a few weeks. But she is still around now, and it's been five months. She has stomach cancer, so she cannot ingest any food. Parts of her intestines were removed, so the only food option for her is intravenous feeding. The doctors know that can only keep you alive for a few weeks. But I gave her the wheatgrass juice through the rectum, which absorbs it into the lymph, and from there to the liver, and it eventually reaches the blood. It essentially feeds the patient. I give 20 ounces total per day, in 3 sessions per day. I also bathe her in the grass. The capillary blood vessels of the skin absorb it and eventually it makes its way into the bloodstream. Most stage five cancer patients die of starvation. But this never happens–not if you're feeding wheatgrass.

Bone, Thyroid, & Skin Problems, Cancer

—Cathleen Peters, Dog Breeder, Welsh Terrier. Youngsville, North Carolina, USA

I breed Welsh Terriers. It's a small business. But I initially got wheatgrass for myself. I was buying it at my local health food store and juicing it myself. So, at some point I just started sharing it with my dogs. I have a sixteen year old Welsh Terrier. He's an old dog. He is quite weak and does not have the energy to run and play outside. I figured it (wheatgrass) couldn't hurt him. Anyway, when he was younger, he always used to go out and chew on the grass.

He liked the wheatgrass juice I fed him, but it was a lot of work to prepare and if I didn't use it right away, the tray would get moldy. Then I found out about the freeze-dried wheatgrass juice (powder). I thought this would be an easier form to use for my dog.

It all started because the dog was old and he had severe problems with his back and with his skin. My vet suspects he has some cancer going on, but we never did a biopsy because at his age, there is no chemo or surgery treatment possible.

So I was taking him once a month to the chiropractor. He was in so much pain that occasionally I even had to give him steroids, but his liver could not handle the steroids. Also, his thyroid was not producing enough thyroid hormone. So we ended up putting him on thyroid medication. Then I realized I needed to do something to regenerate his liver. So I started giving him some of the wheatgrass I was juicing. Later I switched to the wheatgrass powder and mixed it in with apple juice. Things started to improve. I'm not a scientist so I can't tell you that the juice is responsible for everything that happened. But I can tell you this–Welsh Terriers are black with a lot of rich reddish-tan hair. He had lost the red. He had a washed out look. I guess because of his liver problems. But since we started the wheatgrass juice, he's gotten a lot of his color back. Also, the thyroid meds–I don't know whether it was the wheatgrass juice or what–but he needs a lot less of that (thyroid meds), too. I don't know if the wheatgrass juice kicked his body into high-gear or what, but it certainly is a likely possibility.

He's better mentally, too. He had gotten all mixed up. Sleeping during the day and going outside at night. That happens sometimes with older dogs. He's seventeen years old now. The longest one I know of is nineteen, and that is very unusual. He is very frail now. But since putting him on wheatgrass, it seems his body has readjusted to a normal day and night routine. I don't expect that he has much longer, but he definitely improved on the wheatgrass.

This past summer and fall he was able to go out for walks again, which was pretty good for such an old dog with his illness. He really loved the wheatgrass juice. We have always joked about how he would go out and eat grass. Not so much in his old age, but he was definitely drawn to the grass.

Pregnancy and Nursing

The other thing I want to tell you is that we just had a litter of puppies this winter. During the bitch's entire pregnancy and nursing period, I was giving her wheatgrass juice. It is usually hard to keep weight on the mother, but not this time. She actually had lots of milk, and lots of weight. After she weaned the puppies off, I actually had to put her on a diet. That is not typical. I mean, to thrive like that during pregnancy and nursing... You just don't get fat when your body has such a drain on it. I was talking with other Welch Terrier breeders, and everybody agrees how rare it is that she thrived while nursing puppies. I can't swear that it was the wheatgrass, but it had to be, because it was the only thing I did that was different. And the same thing happened in two previous litters, with different bitches. I mean...there's no placebo effect with animals. The puppies were nice and fat and healthy, too. And they're all drinking wheatgrass juice. They initially lapped at it a little and left it. But, now they can't get enough of it. They love it!

You should go to the dog shows and tell them about wheatgrass. If they only knew what this could do, it could be tremendous.

Breast Cancer
—Anne-Marie Baker, Ft. Meyers, Florida

On March 1 of 1996 I had a needle biopsy which, when the results came in, confirmed breast cancer. My doctor recommended an immediate radical mastectomy and a full program of chemotherapy and radiation. I'm a registered nurse. As part of my job, I am in and out of hospitals and doctors offices all the time. So I am well aware of the effects of cancer and the results of the treatment. But I just could not go through with it. So I went against doctor's orders. My colleagues were mortified. First, they were truly concerned for my well being and wondered if I was mentally all there. Secondly, they didn't understand how I could go against the system in which I worked. Some said that I was afraid of how I would look, but that had nothing to do with it. I have seen people go through this therapy hundreds of times and I just don't feel in my heart of hearts that it is the right choice for me. I would never steer anyone away from conventional treatment if that's what they choose. I respect everybody's choice and it is my job to support them in that choice. But for me, I just could not go through with it. Philosophically, I feel it's the wrong approach—destroying all the good cells along with the cancer cells. I want to strengthen my immune system, not debilitate it. After all, if the immune system was strong enough in the first place, the cancer would not have grown. Depressing it [immune system] even more makes it an even harder fight.

So, I was recommended to a holistic doctor who was actually a chiropractor with an extended practice. He worked closely with me in developing a nutritional program that included wheatgrass, raw vegetable juices, supplements, exercise, and detox. For a few months, I was really bombarding this thing pretty intensively. I started out with 1–2 ounces of grass juice, then gradually built up to 6–9 oz. [orally]. I was also doing lots of cleansing through diet, enemas and colon hydrotherapy. After every colonic, my therapist would put in 4 oz. of wheatgrass juice. I would hold that for several hours and I'd say about half of it was absorbed. Then I would do my own enemas daily along with the 4 oz. implants using a bulb syringe. And of course, lots of raw juices during the day—at least 4 juices of 8–12 oz. each. I juiced everything–lots of greens, lots of garlic, sprouts–mostly organic veggies except when I couldn't get them.

Most of my friends are physicians and nurses and at first they told me, "You're in denial," but now they're hushed. You know, since that time, I never called in sick. Not once! I have a better attendance record than anyone in my office.

Since I started the wheatgrass I have more energy than when I was cheerleading in highschool! It's holistic, of course. Exercise is a big part of it too, and I do lots of yoga. Now I'm on a regular routine at a more relaxed pace. I'm working a full time job with a lot of running around. I had an AMASS test six months ago and it came up negative. No sign of cancer, anywhere! I have a lot of confidence in what I'm doing. I think it's important to surround yourself with positive supportive people. Otherwise you're fighting a double fight, battling with the outer world as well as the inner one. You just don't need to raise the odds. Besides, you learn a lot from supportive people. Everybody you meet either gives you a boost or a knock. You've got to change your lifestyle. I'm glad I have the flexibility to run home and make a juice. My health is more important than my job. If you don't change the [lifestyle] circumstances which led to the problem then I don't care if you cut it, burn it, or poison it, it will come back.

I don't think there is one answer to cancer or health. It's an accumulation of a whole bunch of different therapies. But wheatgrass was fundamental to my therapy. I read that it's the abscisic acid [a naturally occurring compound that has both inhibitory and promoting functions] in wheatgrass that targets the cancer cells. I just wish I could sneak a juicer into the hospital and make wheatgrass for all my patients.

Bladder Cancer
—Dorothy Naylor, Naples, Florida

What can I say? I'm supposed to be dead according to them. My bladder was totally covered with tumors. Now, my MRI doesn't show any. None. My bladder was cut so many times and lasered and scraped and fried. Then the chemotherapy, the radiation, all the drugs. It was awful. It fried the surface of my bladder. And during that whole time, whenever I would go back for an examination, there would always be another tumor or two. The MRI and sonogram always showed up some new cancers. I had them removed at least six times. The doctor was always scraping them out and cutting them out. So he says, "We can't do this forever–let's remove it." He wants to remove the bladder. That's his solution, surgery. Then I'd have a tube and a bag hanging out....that's awful. But I didn't have any alternatives, at that time. So I went into the operating room and right there, just before they were going to take it out, I had a heart attack on the table. It wasn't severe, but it was enough to stop the surgery.

That heart attack saved my life. You see the doctor told me and my family that I wouldn't last long enough to visit my children in August. This was April. My son was furious with him. I didn't feel like I was going to die. It was at that point, I decided to look for alternatives. I wasn't going to let them remove my bladder and no more laser or scraping the tumors, either. I had enough.

My daughter from Germany got me started on wheatgrass. No one else in the family knew about it but her. I have 13 children, you know. With her help, I started drinking wheatgrass everyday. I was religious about it. My children got me a Green Power juicer. I like it but it's a lot to clean. Then I started growing my own wheatgrass, but I just couldn't do that. That was too hard. Now, I get it right down the street. Back then, I got it shipped in for $8/lb. At one point I took as much as 7 ounces of grass juice per day. But then, my body couldn't tolerate it, so now I'm back down to 6 ounces per day. Two ounces in the morning, 2 in the afternoon and 2 in the evening.

It's been 4 years now, and I only had one tumor since because I was visiting my daughter and I was neglectful. I went off the wheatgrass. When I got home I had a tumor! Well, I've never left the program since then and there has never been another tumor. My MRI and sonogram are clean. My bladder is not a problem anymore. My doctor—he's nice, but strictly conventional—says: "Just keep doing what you're doing."

Candidiasis, Irritable Bowel, Leaky Gut Syndrome

Tony Gentile of Malaga NJ is a former collegiate wrestler and teacher who had to quit his job because of complications from irritable bowel and leaky gut syndrome.

My problems started during my wrestling years. Because we had to meet the weight requirements I was on a fiberless diet because fiber adds weight. So I'd have two candy bars for dinner and get false energy from that instead of eating real food. I also got dehydrated because water was a no-no—it adds weight. The competition years ruined my health by starving my body for nutrition and killing my intestines without fiber or water. I had chronic constipation and dehydration and became dependent on laxatives. That was the start of my digestion problems. From there I developed candidiasis, leaky gut syndrome and eventually arthritis. My knees got so bad I had two operations on them and they still are [many years later] weak and painful. My intestinal condition was so debilitating I couldn't focus at work. I quit my job.

I've been fighting this fight for 20 years, now. I've tried everything; nothing works. Only wheatgrass has helped me. The implants are great. I do an enema first to clear myself out and to better hold the implant. I take 6 ounces of [wheatgrass] juice mixed with about 2 ounces of aloe vera gel and a little warm water. Making it body temperature helps retain it better. I put it [all] in an enema bag and attach the 12 inch tube. [A 12 inch enema extension catheter is available by special order from your pharmacy.] I get on the slant board with feet high to get it as far in as possible so it reaches the portal vein and goes to the liver. I let it slowly leak in, real slow and hold it for as long as possible, ideally 30 minutes. In 2 minutes the burning [irritable bowel] is gone and I'm feeling high. Since I've been doing wheatgrass, my digestion is ten times better. My hair got thicker, the white spots left my nails, the dark rings around my eyes cleared up and the pain in my legs is gone. There is a change in my muscle quality, too. They're firmer; my knees last much longer.

After 20 days of implants, 6 ounces each twice per day with the extension tube, that fire [of pain] in my colon was gone. I mean gone. My liver is not swelled up anymore. That hardness, it's not there, gone. Not sure why, but you're getting really high assimilation of a complete food. Then you have the implants purging the liver and cleaning the blood. I can feel it. The blood feeds the muscles, ligaments and tendons. It's the chlorophyll. It's just healing and cleansing. Did you read that chlorophyll book by [Dr. Bernard] Jensen? It's the enzymes, too. They're catalysts. My digestion is 100% better. I take a couple of shots [15-20 minutes] before I eat. It gets my cylinders firing. My irritable bowel...it's the only thing that has helped me. I'm growing tons of sunflower and buckwheat [sprouts] now, too. I make lots of blended drinks [with them]. My candida and my digestion are 100% better. I sleep better at night, too....less of that AM toxicity when I wake up.

—

Wheatgrass contains raw chlorophyll. Chlorophyll is condensed sunlight. Since we are light beings, spirit and soul inside solid bodies, the light force vibrates through the physical body. That's the energy you feel. Wheatgrass is a spiritual food. It nourishes you on a spiritual level as well as the physical.
—Piter U. Caizer, The Wheatgrass Messiah

Grass and Marathon Endurance

—Bruce McVay, Salt Lake City, Utah[1]

The newspapers have recently published several articles on animal studies that have proved that very low calorie, highly nutritional diets enhance strength, endurance and longevity. Wheatgrass has by lab analysis proven to be very close to, if not the foremost plant in the category of nutritive value per ounce. Being an ultra–distance runner for five years [races from thirty to one hundred miles or more], I tried every physically enhancing supplement and natural food source to improve my health, stamina, and oxygenation process. One and one-half years ago, I began juicing one to six ounces of grass juice daily. After one to two months of cleansing—which consisted of a few headaches and itching—I began to notice tremendous changes in my performance, energy, stamina, etc. Always in the past, I was a middle to rear of the pack racer. Wheatgrass changed that.

This year, I ran a twenty-six mile race in the Teton Mountains and won by half an hour. This race was at the top of the Tetons, 12,000 to 13,000 feet high, and down to Jackson Hole, Wyoming. Ultra distance runners from all over the United States participated. At the eighteen mile checkpoint, some people with twice the amount of training as me quit the race. Two or three finished. Something I noticed was that I never hit the wall (nausea, etc.) like I had sometimes in previous races. I was exhilarated all the way to the end of the race.

On June 5, I participated in an eleven and one-half hour hour run-a-thon at the Utah State Prison. I ran over sixty-two miles eating primarily wheat and barley grass mixed with fresh apple juice. During this time, I expended over 6,500 calories. My nearest competitor was ten miles behind. These are factual examples, but the best result is the way I feel all the time and during the race—very comfortable under physical and mental stress.

Some people would think that I increased my training or trained long and hard for these races, but in reality, I cut my training in half during this period of time. I had cut my training mileage from sixty to ninety miles per week to thirty to forty miles per week. Imagine! Less training, but better performance!

I have broken most of my own personal records. Another thing that amazed me about the prison race, was that my laps at the last of the race were as fast as the laps at the beginning. Wheatgrass helps numerous processes in the body, but improved oxygenation [enhanced oxygen absorption] is the best one. I believe in it.

Colon, Lymph and Liver Cancer
—*Gary Garrett, Gainesville, Florida*

In June 1995 I was told that I had a large tumor in my colon. Dr. Wyshbaum my oncologist, told me I had only one option: have immediate surgery to remove a section of the colon. I followed this advice and had the surgery.

The doctor then told me the tumor was approximately the size of a baseball and had grown through the colon wall to adjoining tissue and the cancer had metastasized to six lymph nodes and my liver. The prognosis was not very good. They expected further tumor activity within one year. My surgeon strongly recommended that I have surgery on the liver and begin a course of radiation of the lymph system and chemotherapy for the colon as soon as possible. Before I could even consider this I began to have complications from the surgery: the incision would not close up. It required new dressings three times a day for the eighteen days I was hospitalized, and for months after I was sent home. As long as my wound would not heal I could not have any toxic chemo or radiation. After surgery I could not have anything by mouth–even water–for twelve days, only IV's.

It was during this time that a good friend found out I was sick, contacted my wife and offered his assistance. He had been fighting a similar battle with cancer for some time. He has read many books and done much research on his own. He gained valuable information which he was willing to share with me. This included diet changes and learning all about something called wheatgrass. As I mentioned earlier, my wound required dressing three times daily. Even with strong pain killers like morphine it was almost unbearable to have the nurses wrap and unwrap the area so often. After 12 days on IV's I could finally begin to take liquids by mouth. I first experienced wheatgrass juice when a friend brought 6 ounces to my hospital room, which I drank right down. I didn't notice anything until the next day when my morning nurse came to dress my wound. As I mentioned, it became so painful I dreaded these times. What a pleasant surprise the next day when my nurse began to take the dressing off and I could tolerate it because it was not as sensitive as before. Then an amazing thing happened, the nurse pulled out the packing and we both noticed it had turned green.

At first this scared her because they are trained to watch for changes in the dressings. When they are green it usually means a very serious infection. However, I had told the nurse about the wheatgrass and she recognized that the color change was a result of the chlorophyll. Imagine my surprise that in one day of drinking crude, dark green chlorophyll, it passed through my entire system and finds its way to this external wound and reduces my pain.

As time went by, my home care nurses were amazed at how quickly my wound healed. The wound packing continued to have a green tint throughout the whole time. When I left the hospital I was so weak I could hardly climb a flight of stairs. But by taking wheatgrass juice daily, in a matter of weeks, I was able to return to a full work schedule with no new tumor growth in my colon.

The following was written by Mrs. Gary (Kathleen) Garrett, July 1998.

Gary had colon cancer and six lymph cancers and one spot on the liver. Dr. Botonay heavily insisted on chemo and radiation. I asked him "If we did all that, would we get rid of the cancer?" He said it would give Gary six more months. Gary and I left his office determined to seek alternatives. Why poison the immune system if you're trying to strengthen it? I'm an X-ray technician and Mom is a nurse. We saw what wheatgrass was doing for Gary even though we never had a drop of it. I thought it was a joke at first; now I'm a total believer. Half of his incision reopened and we watched the grass heal it. That was amazing, and wheatgrass kept the cancer out, too. It never came back to the colon–it never came back to the lymph, and the liver tumor had completely calcified. Gary's CEA [carcinoembryonic antigen test] was only at 40. It should have been in the hundreds or thousands with cancer as advanced as his. His was incredibly low. We had the cancer beat. Even the bone scans and other tests proved that it never went into bone or the lungs or anywhere else. But the calcified remains of the tumor on the liver obstructed his bile so they put a tube in his side to drain the bile. That caused a bad infection. He was hospitalized sixteen times between April and December. They kept redoing the tube and reinfecting the liver and the infection traveled throughout his whole body. His body started to shut down. He wasn't able to make his own platelets. A normal platelet count is 150,000. Gary's was at 61,000. You start hemorrhaging when you're that low. We don't take blood transfusions; we're Jehovah Witness'. We needed to raise the platelets without a transfusion. All our hopes turned to wheatgrass. Dr. Smith [cancer surgeon] permitted us to give 2 oz of wheatgrass every 4 hours through a tube down his nose that went directly into his small intestine. My son Kenny and I grew it, juiced it, and gave it to him. Everyday we watched his platelet count rise. There was no question about it. They took a blood work up every day. It's fully documented. But Gary was in septic shock from the infection. He was too ill even to raise a fever.

Gary's platelets rose every day for seven days. From 61,000 to 141,000 strictly from the wheatgrass, nothing else. It's all documented through the lab work. How could someone that ill, with his immune system and his kidneys both shut down, make such a comeback nearly reaching normal blood count? Dr. Smith called it a medical phenomenon. Now, he's taking wheatgrass!

Gary didn't make it. But he lived 3 years despite Dr. Wyshbaum's prognosis of 6 months. Gary had a friend in Pennsylvania with colon cancer and was also given six months. He went through the recommended chemo and radiation and died in 6 months anyway. Gary spent 3 years on wheatgrass working 16 hour days. Despite his excess weight—he was over 300 lbs.—Gary was running up and down stairs and in between he ran back to the hospital to get intravenous antibiotics for the infection they [the doctors] induced. His energy was remarkable. He was back to work 10 times faster than they predicted. He took 4–8 ounces of juice every day, both orally and by implants. He held those implants in all day sometimes. We went to another hospital for five weeks and I didn't have any wheatgrass there. His immune system wasn't able to counter the toxic overload. He was getting thinner and weaker. It was the double whammy of the hospital induced liver infection in a critical organ, and the toxic overload that overcame his immune system. If I only had wheatgrass during those five weeks away from home, it could have made all the difference.

In Gary's honor, his wife Kathleen and sons continue to grow wheatgrass for people in their area and beyond. (See Resources: Wheatgrass Express.)

Senior Citizen on Grass Out-Lifts Bodybuilders
—Leland Bender, Bloomingdale, Illinois.

My son Eddie at age 51 was ready to die. He smoked for 30 years—3–4 packs every day since he was 18. He weighed 315 pounds and couldn't walk a hundred feet without gasping for breath. Doc said, "You got plugged arteries." He was only 50 years old! But he was not ready to die. I got him on the wheatgrass program. Steve, listen to me—you cannot believe the turnaround in him. He did wheatgrass juice every day; he lost 50 lbs; he dropped the meat 100%. He's eating sprouts. Evidently wheatgrass does rejuvenate the lungs, because now he can trot right along with the rest of us. He's feeling great.

And I'll tell you what, he's not going back to work. Not the same work. We're going into the wheatgrass business. Father and son. We're calling it NutriGrow. We're going to supply gyms and individuals with the growing materials via network marketing. It's gonna explode. It's got to. You wanna hear a story? Call Addison Gold's gym [Bloomingdale, IL]; speak to Mike Niewinski, the manager. Ask him about wheatgrass. He'll tell you. He won't be without it. We can't grow it fast enough for him. I got the grow racks in there with lights and automatic misters. We sold over 300 trays of grass and 50 juicers. The guys in the gym are going ape over the stuff. They don't need steroids anymore. They feel an energy surge within 15–20 minutes. The bloodstream just sucks that nutrition right in. Just sucks it in. They lift another 20%. That's the edge on the competition. I'm telling you, it's going to explode. And they need your sprouts, too. Pea sprouts, broccoli sprouts, sunflower, buckwheat. Your sprout bags are great.

It's just amazing stuff. In the past year I've walked in excess of 700 miles across Illinois. I do 2–3 miles per day everyday in all weather. I'm telling you it's the wheatgrass. I can't believe my strength. I'll be seventy-two on November 24th. I've had cardiovascular strength before, but now...I go on the spin cycle for an hour without stopping. There's an instructor putting us through the paces. The young ones are dropping out after 20 minutes. But I roll through a full solid hour without gasping for breath. And my strength! My trainer will tell you, I out-lift in endurance 70% of the gym regardless of their age. And we work hard. One and a half, two hours, I mean the perspiration just rolls off of you. And I don't have a sore spot on my body. I'm as flexible now as when I was eighteen. And my weight—I lost forty lbs. I'm 235 now. I was 275. It definitely eliminates the hunger.

Yeah, I tried the powder. You don't get the same effect. Common sense will tell you, it's gotta be live. You can feel an energy surge within 15 minutes. I grow my grass usually five to six inches for eight or so days. It's a real rich green. I'm up to six ounces per day, now. [Drinking] Three in the morning; three in the evening. No antacids any more, whatsoever. Chlorophyll—that's the best antacid.

You know, I've had a kind of gravel in my voice for years. I chalked it up to age. People over fifty have a lot of phlegm. After two weeks on wheatgrass I spit up plugs of phlegm. Gone. It's gone! You can hear my voice echoing. I told the doc, he says, "No wonder, it's all clean in there."

I've been through the hospital system. I had advanced gout. Too much meat. I mean this is the old days, of course. Now my former hematologist is on alfalfa tablets and is about to come into the wheatgrass program. He actually lost weight. It definitely takes care of that gnawing feeling of hunger. You're empty, but satisfied.

And there's another miracle, too. Mike's father-in-law—his fingers were always tingling and then they would go numb. This was going on for 2 solid years. Mike walks into the gym and he says: 'Lee, you cured my father-in-law. No more pain; no more tingling in his fingers.' It's two months later, still no numbing, no tingling, no pain.

I'll tell you what. After they get rid of the cigarettes, they should outlaw McDonald's and Burger King. I mean, how many generations do we have to sicken before they figure it out. We can't afford to pay for it anymore. The insurance companies are way out of line. The people can't pay. The sick are just going to wind up on public aid. That's the way it's gonna be. And that goes for the nursing homes, too. Half the people in there didn't have to be if they had just done a better job on their exercise and nutrition. I'll tell you where the problem begins–it's the kids. "Mommy I want french fries–I want pretzels...chocolate." Only 1% of the kids have good nutrition. They get away with it because of the TV. It hypnotizes them. I'll tell you what, we gotta get this stuff on Oprah Winfrey. It's all about the media. That's all it will take. But one way or the other, the word will come out. It has to. This stuff is too incredible.

—

Never Underestimate the Power of Nature

Grass and Melanoma
—Neva Whetzel, Singers Glen, Virginia

I noticed a small mole had begun to grow. It was about ¼ inch. I checked it out with my kinesiologist who is really great and we determined it was cancerous. I went to see a specialist who diagnosed it as a melanoma and gave me a "one in a million" chance of survival. He was adamant that it be surgically removed including all surrounding tissue. He wanted to remove a 3x5 area going down into the muscle and also remove my lymph nodes. It was in the upper thigh area. Then he would graft skin back on. He wanted me on a full chemotherapy and radiation program. This was only a ¼ inch melanoma mind you. The only thing I would let him do was remove the quarter inch spot. No more. Then I went on the wheatgrass.

I have been eating well all along—I am not a junk food person. So I went back to my kinesiologist and we checked out what to do for it and that's when I started the wheatgrass. Actually any kind of grass checked out good–barley, Kamut–even the powdered grasses tested fine. I took those whenever I was without the fresh. Several herbs checked out good as well and I took those too. I did lots of things. You can't say it was just the wheatgrass.

I started growing the fresh grass in my backyard in the spring. I grew it in the ground and let it mature [to the jointing stage]. I would fast for 10 days at a time and repeat that a few times. I drank 8 ounces at a time—I'm an all or nothing person. Sometimes it would nauseate me and I'd get dizzy from it—probably a liver reaction from dumping toxins. But we had a lot of wheatgrass and we wanted to use it up because it's no good unless it's fresh. So my husband Dennis drank it, too. We both took 8 oz of wheatgrass on an empty stomach over the course of one hour. That's how I took it. One thing I noticed after a while, my hair softened. It just got soft, like a baby's hair. My facial skin felt soft, too. What a reaction. I couldn't figure out where it was coming from unless it was the grass. But what really amazed me was that Dennis had the same response. His hair was silkier, too! And it wasn't like we even told each other about it. It just happened.

Well, I went back to the same doctor a year and a half later and do you know what he said, "I was really worried about you. Apparently what we did for you in the office that day cured you."

Slipped Disk Dog, Lyme Disease, Emotions
— *Loreta Vainius, Malvern Pennsylvania.*

My dog Spirgis is a long haired mini dachshund. When he was only 4 years old, he got really, really sick. He had a high fever; he could not move or do anything. He was defecating wherever he sat. His eyes were murky. He was definitely dying. I took him to the vet. They gave him steroids and antibiotics. A friend recommended a veterinary chiropractor who discovered Spirgis had a slipped disk. He gave him an adjustment but when he tested him by pinching him between the toes, there was no feeling. Spirgis didn't respond at all. The doctor said that it had gone too far and there was nothing he could do. He suggested a veterinary surgeon. So I went to this veterinary surgeon and I said, "Is there anything you can do? He's got a slipped disk and he's paralyzed." The surgeon says, "There is a possibility we might be able to do something, but it's not very certain." He told me the operation would cost $1,800 and there was no guarantee. He told me, if he still can't walk, they would make a little wheel for him to roll on.

Well, it took me a while to learn to use my own therapy [she uses wheatgrass and gives it to others]. I mean, how do you give a dog an enema? I figured, what did I have to lose? It was a good thing it was summer! I gave him 4 enemas in five days. We did it outside on a table. It took three of us to give the dog an enema. First I gave him a coffee enema followed by a tray of grass [eight-ten ounces]. After the fourth implant he shifted his body. He couldn't go anywhere of course but it was an indication that he was responding. Then I got an eyedropper and held his snout and I put two ounces of grass right into his mouth. Two in the morning and two in the evening, every day. It took me fifteen minutes to get it into him. About thirty minutes later he would throw it up. It was a very slimy and heavy mucous. He kept on vomiting. We did this all outside. Then I realized–he was throwing up the toxins! After two weeks, my cousin came over with his two dogs and Spirgis started running around like crazy, dragging his hind legs all around. What a sight. This dog had a slipped disk, he had a tumor in his neck and a pinched vertebrae. None of the doctors had any hope. I mean, this is a miracle dog!

I continued this for five weeks: wheatgrass in the morning and wheatgrass in the evening. Remember he was dragging his hind legs. The muscles were atrophied. We had to tie socks on them to protect them. Then, after the fifth week of giving him wheatgrass morning and evening, Spirgis got up, lifted his hind leg and started to walk. Eventually, he came with me on my [jogging] runs. He was healed completely. The vet could not believe this dog was still alive.

But that's just one story. In 1994, I got lyme disease. I actually got it in April but we didn't realize what it was until I was diagnosed in August. I felt like I had a huge hole in the pit of my stomach. I mean it didn't matter if I ate ten pounds of food, I couldn't fill it. Later I learned that it's an emotional need that cannot be filled by food. But one night I stuffed myself with corn chips and apples and fruit and candy. Then I went to the Olive Garden, ate two salads and a plate of pasta. I was desperately trying to fill the hole in my stomach. I had to drive two hours so I drank Coca-Cola to keep awake. When I got home that night I started to throw up. I threw up fifteen times, continuously. I was white as a sheet. I was completely off balance; the room started to spin. I was totally out of electrolytes. I told my friend, "Get me some warm water and juice a tray of wheatgrass." I put eight ounces of wheatgrass into a 1,000ml enema bag of filtered water. And I did it again and again–three times. It took me an hour and a half. I put it in and held 2,750ml total of water and three trays of grass in my colon and by the time I put the last tray in, I could see the color coming back into my body. It started at my feet and you could literally see it rising up. In any other circumstance I would have been bedridden for days. But eighteen hours later I was out keeping my appointments and I felt absolutely alive.

When I feel tension and nervousness and emotional upheaval that I can't deal with, I take a wheatgrass enema and I come out a brand new person. I really feel I'm reversing the whole aging process. If I had not healed the emotional stuff, I'm sure it would have gone into a tumor or cancer. Wheatgrass is my miracle drug.

My husband takes Green Magma [barley grass juice powder] regularly. I don't. I only take it fresh; I like my home grown. I don't drink it at all. I just do my enemas. I could be working an entire day and be exhausted. I come home and I find my wheatgrass healing and cleansing and energizing. It's a powerful, powerful food.

Cancer of the Throat, Alimentary Canal and Melanoma
—Ruth Williams of Smyrna, Georgia

Words in italics are that of Mr. Eugene Williams, husband

Let me relate a long, complicated, and painful experience in just a few words. In 1961, I had a cancerous mole excised from my toe. Like the tree with its trunk being removed, the root system evidently remained. By 1976 my body was saturated with cancer. The melanoma had metastasized. It was in my throat and my alimentary canal. I could barely talk and it was impossible for me to take solid food.

[Mr. Eugene Williams] *She was comatose and whittled down to only 62 lbs. We were in and out of five hospitals. She had chemotherapy and radiation. She was in an isolation room. Before I would go into to see her I had to shower and put on special clothing. Every vital life sign was gone. There was no possibility of living according to the medical doctors. They told me, "Be prepared. It could be a very short time."*

I did not want to stay in the hospital. I dropped down and prayed that the Lord would take me home. They sent me home to die with terminal cancer.

A neighbor of mine said, "You don't have to die," and gave me a book called *How I Conquered Cancer Naturally* by Eydie Mae. With the aid of my nurse, we began growing and juicing wheatgrass and I started taking multiple wheatgrass enemas and implants daily. To keep up with this I had to grow 10 trays of wheatgrass daily. After a few weeks on this schedule, I had my first major healing crisis. I vomited continuously and it was awful, but I had faith in God.

Slowly, but perceptibly, I began to notice improvement. I was able to take small amounts of nourishment by mouth. Gradually, I increased the wheatgrass to 10 ounces per implant. Just six months after I started the wheatgrass program, I was able to walk again.

My situation was still severe and recovery was very slow over a long period of time. I got help from some very special doctors including Ann Wigmore whom I visited at her institute in Boston three times. As the raw food intake increased, I was able to reduce the frequency of the implants. In the years that followed I returned to normal weight.

It's 22 years later now, Ruth will soon be 75. She still uses wheatgrass and you should see her...in spite of where she has been, she is a picture of health.

I am alive and well. The Lord Jesus Christ spared my life. I am grateful to God for showing me the healing power of wheatgrass.

Lymphatic Cancer
—by Dennis Lampro, Chicago, Illinois

I was in school taking an airline computer course when I began to feel very tired and draggy. I began to lose weight, so I went to the doctor who did a lot of tests and couldn't find what was wrong. I noticed my lymph nodes were getting bigger and bigger, so they did more testing and found that I had lymphatic cancer which was spreading throughout my body.

The doctors began treating me with certain drugs which didn't work because I was sensitive to them. The cancer was getting worse and worse and they put me on chemotherapy. At this point, they gave me three months to live if I took the therapy. All my hair fell out, and I got big blisters because my immune system was destroyed.

Right about that time a lady told me about wheatgrass, which I had never heard of. I had never heard of live foods and I never ate salads. I was a *McDonalds* person. She started bringing me wheatgrass and I began drinking the juice.

She also taught me to meditate to help with the pain. The doctors had me on morphine, but with meditation I stopped taking pain medication. I also realized that the lymph nodes were getting smaller. At that point I was directed to do a fast with wheatgrass juice.

I was very nauseous and had diarrhea. I was really cleansing. Then I went up to 2 ounces in 4 separate doses a day with distilled water in between and nothing else. I did that for thirty days and within that time my lymphatic system became completely clean. It took a bit longer to become normal, but the size of the nodes became normal. After that I added a variety of sprouts including sunflower and buckwheat and learned more about the diet from the Hippocrates books.[2]

The implants were interesting because that was where I got the pain relief. If I was in a lot of pain, I would get up and do an implant and within 45 minutes to an hour the pain was bearable. The wheatgrass juice implants also made it easier for me to breathe because the chemotherapy generated a lot of mucus in my lungs. It took about 3 months to get rid of it.

My thoughts were clearer. I was coughing up lots of mucus. In fact, this near-death experience actually introduced me to a whole spiritual world that I had no idea existed. I was enriched as a person. It took six months before the illness left completely. Six months ago my doctor tested me and could find nothing wrong.

It runs in my family to become gray early, but my gray hair disappeared. I could hardly believe it. My mother thought I was plucking the gray out. No way! At age thirty-one, I look and feel younger than I ever have before.

—

I'm not going to no doctor. Last time I went to the doctor, he
gave me so much medicine, I was sick long after I got well.
     —Chico Marx, 'Horse Feathers'

Prostate Cancer
—Bill Nasdy, Bonita Springs, Florida

I had prostate cancer; my PSA [prostate specific antigen] was fourteen–the lowest it's ever been was five. At first, I agreed to the surgery–major surgery to remove the whole prostate. This is February; the operation was scheduled for May. I also agreed to a program of intensive chemo and radiation. I'm seventy [years old] but I'm fit. First they put me on Flutamide. You know what that is? I found out later it's a chemical castrator. It was awful—the worst stuff. It sucked all the energy right out of me.

I went to a support group and somebody told me about wheatgrass. I went out and bought *The Wheatgrass Book* by Wigmore. Right then, I decided to stop the treatment and went full speed into natural therapy. I canceled the surgery and got off the drug after 5 weeks of that hell. I changed everything. They told me, "You're going against doctor's orders." Well, I've become a vegetarian now which is a big deal for me because I grew up in meat country. Right away my PSA went down. (I test it every month.) I'm taking six to eight ounces a day [wheatgrass]. I take it before every meal. It's changed my whole life. I'm also taking ozone therapy at the Optimum Institute in Naples. It's fantastic, and they don't even charge for it. And I'm pouring on the antioxidants, too—Essiac tea, CQ10, shark liver oil, vitamin E, saw palmetto and 9,000mg of vitamin C daily. Antioxidants is the way to go and wheatgrass is, of course, loaded with them.

You know I forgot to tell you, four years ago I had microwave treatment done on my prostate to relieve painful urination. It was not successful at all and I strongly believe it had a lot to do with creating the cancer. It wasn't approved by the FDA then but it's accepted both here and in Canada now. I would never do that again and I definitely don't recommend it. This is the trouble with the medical establishment. They let you take damaging treatments even before they're officially approved and then they approve them, while nontoxic wheatgrass and ozone are outlawed. We've got to take back control of our health from the government and the doctors. They're not gods. It's unbelievable that the public trusts them the way they do. They're pushing dangerous drugs and dangerous therapies and unnecessary surgery. I mean c'mon, this is nuts! But the tide is turning. The middle class is getting on the bandwagon. Look at me, I never knew about this stuff!

I'm in remission now. On my last PSA test which is the newest type of PSA...the nurse says to me, "I hope you didn't do any exercise today." I had just come from doing 50 laps in the pool! Turns out exercise artificially elevates the PSA. I said "Hell, fifty-eight bucks down the drain!" Guess what? I got a call the next day, my PSA was 0.12.

Listen, I'm an active guy for my age, but I was dragging. You wanna know what the real surprise for me was? Since the wheatgrass, I've got twice as much energy. I sky dive; I work a full time job; I swim 50 laps. And let me tell you, it's all about exercise and diet. Your immune system will take care of you if you take care of it. That's the key. And you can't do it if you're bombarding yourself with smoking and drinking and bad food and high stress and toxic drugs. Chemotherapy kills the cancer but as soon as you stop, bang!–it comes right back somewhere else and it's worse.

I got eight trays of wheatgrass growing right now and I wanna tell you something else. Since I've started this, I've never had a cold, never had the flu. My wife was sick but I never caught it. Cuts and sores heal up immediately; it has definitely changed my life. I also take a carrot juice every day with garlic—lots of garlic—beets, parsley and sprouts, lots of sprouts, in the salad especially. No dairy, no beef, no pork, no chicken—the only thing I'll take is a deep sea fish occasionally. I'm a believer in it [vegetarianism]. Give me the grains and vegetables; give me the grass instead of waiting for the cow to eat it and then eating the cow.

Lupus, Hysterectomy
—Cynthia Gebhart, Geneva, Florida

I have lupus—I don't know if you know what that is? It's when the antibodies in your blood start attacking your normal cells. The symptoms are everywhere. I get rashes on my skin, my joints swell up, headaches, shortness of breath, real flu-like symptoms, depression...I just feel lethargic all the time. I'm a real active person, too. Ask anyone–I'm always in motion. I got a full time job. I help my husband out. I got two kids; we live on the St. Johns River. But this lupus just lays me flat on my back and anything can trigger a bout of it. I'm walking on egg shells most of the time.

A year ago, after I had a root canal, the lupus flared up and wiped me out for months. Two years before that, I had a cyst removed on the right ovary. It took me five months to recover from that. I had such severe pain; I could not get beyond the pain and nothing I did worked. I was tired and run down all the time. My joints swelled, my skin tissue got inflamed. I had the desire to work but not the stamina. So, I was definitely afraid of a hysterectomy. I watched my aunt and my sister both go through it. I sat with them while they moaned and groaned for six months. And they didn't have lupus! So I was paranoid as hell about this surgery.

So I figured before I go under the knife, I gotta try to control the lupus. My husband and I got on the internet and we looked up all the lupus doctors and we picked out the best one. I mean this guy was world renowned, head of his department, a prestigious hospital....the best. So I dragged myself out of bed and we went to Atlanta, Georgia. The doctor examined me and said: You're dying. I want you to go straight to the hospital. When I arrived, they started pumping me full of steroids and two different types of drugs and IV's. Then I *really was* dying! When I got out of that hospital I slept for two weeks. I could not get out of bed and I'm a perpetually active person. My husband kept saying, "You were not this sick before you started all these drugs." So we went back to Atlanta and he checked me again and put me back in the hospital again. I kept on asking him, "Why?" And I never felt like I got a good enough answer. I kept trying to tell my husband, "He never gives me a straight answer." That's not right. He just kept pumping me with more drugs. I was looking and feeling worse. This was another two weeks in the hospital. My husband says, "You were never this ill before; we need to get you off these drugs." By the grace of God, that's when we ran into Russell.[3]

Russell had put my uncle on wheatgrass so I dropped the drugs and decided to give it a try. I used to tease my uncle; I'd moo like a cow. But I wanna tell you, three weeks into drinking the grass juice, and I felt like I could climb Mount Everest. I mean, you have no idea how long it's been since I've felt this good. I felt like I could touch the clouds. My worst fear was that it was a fluke and it would end. Then I started echinacea and ozone. My husband and I were totally flabbergasted by all the wonderful information and therapies we were discovering. And my GP [doctor] could not believe my cholesterol. I'm always testing it because I have this thyroid disorder. It's always been between 240 and 280 for years. All of a sudden it's 173. After the wheatgrass—that's the only thing I did different! Of course, I got off the drugs. He told me, by the way, that I was taking enough antibiotics to kill an elephant. So much for big shot specialists! Now, I take nothing unless it's natural. I'm growing the grass and juicing it and celery and carrots and taking different herbs and I feel great. Yes, I did go through with the surgery, [hysterectomy] and this is the most unbelievable part: Not *only* did I *not* have a lupus flare-up, but in two weeks after that major operation I was back home stripping my bed and cooking food and I haven't stopped since. There is absolutely *no* doubt in my mind that wheatgrass was the thing that turned everything around. I've been through too many operations, too many hospitals, and too much hell for anyone to tell me otherwise.

—

The effect these highly nutritious green drinks are having on all my patients, especially my arthritis patients, is nothing short of amazing... I tell you, no matter what your age or present condition, these grass superfoods can quickly take you to a whole new level of radiant health—sparkling eyes, abundant energy, pain-free joints and a zest for living you remember from the healthiest days of your life. —Dr. Julian Whitaker, MD, editor of Health & Healing Newsletter.[4]

—

As measured by present standards, our diet is better than ever before in history. Yet, we are fighting a losing battle against degenerative diseases. Cancer and heart disease have worsened with every decade and this is in spite of all our knowledge about vitamins and advances in medical science. There is something missing in our diet and it may well be the grass leaf factors. —Dr. Charles F. Schnabel, 1939.[5]

—

The art of healing comes from nature, not from the physician. Therefore the physician must start from nature with an open mind. —Paracelsus, 1493–1541[6]

Wheatgrass Retreats

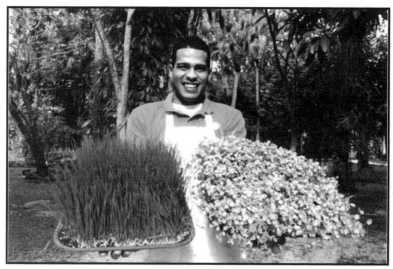

Wheatgrass and Buckwheat greens at the Hippocrates Health Institute, in sunny West Palm Beach, Florida.

Sanctuaries for recuperation from chronic disease and restoration of health have been around for centuries. Hippocrates, the father of modern medicine, is quoted as saying: "Rest is sometimes the best remedy." The Chinese have an ancient adage: "Healing is three parts treatment, seven parts nursing." In modern times, American physician Edward Trudeau became famous for curing tuberculosis at his sanitarium in the fresh air of New York's Adirondack mountains. This was 60 years before the development of the modern drug treatment. John Harvey Kellogg, co-founder of the Kellogg Cereal company, was a prestigious surgeon from Bellevue Hospital Medical College in New York. But he had a passion for nutrition, vegetarianism, and natural hygiene and ran two popular sanitariums in Battle Creek and Miami. The treatments in these places were fresh air, rest, exercise, and healthy diet. When the focus on body, mind and spirit is intensified along with insulation from the stresses of society, miracles happen. Our society places great emphasis on outside appearances— skin, cosmetics, and muscles. If the color of our lungs, the hardness of our livers or the congestion of our colons were visible to all, we would place greater emphasis on keeping our insides in pristine condition. Every middle class family is stretched to their limits paying health insurance bills. But the best insurance of all is a couple of weeks each year at a health retreat where you can cleanse, nourish, rejuvenate, and heal. The following is a list of some of the major training centers worldwide where wheatgrass is a central part of a total holistic lifestyle rejuvenation program. Refer to the *Resources* chapter for additional references.

Hippocrates Health Institute

561-471-8876, fax 561-471-9464. 800-842-2125.
1443 Palmdale Court, West Palm Beach, FL 33411.
www.hippocratesinstitute.com

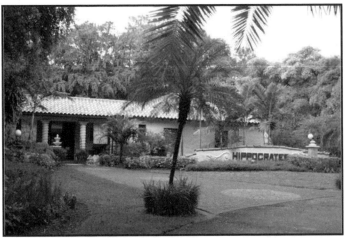

The entrance to Hippocrates, West Palm Beach, Florida.

After my stay at Hippocrates, I continued following the
program strictly. Not only did I eventually get rid of my
malignant breast tumor, I also increased my energy level,
improved my skin tone and hair volume. Most importantly,
I have been cancer-free for nearly a decade now. I return to the
Institute twice a year for reinforcement and reaffirmation.

—Rachel Budnick, Chicago, Illinois

Nestled in the quiet woods of West Palm Beach Florida is an oasis of health and healing where people from all over the globe convene to mend their bodies and revive their selves. This serene thirty-acre sanctuary carries forth and expands upon the visions of Ann Wigmore and Viktoras Kulvinskas who founded the original Hippocrates Health Institute in Boston in the 1960's. Co-directors Anna Maria and Brian Clement both hold NMDs and PhDs in Nutrition. Brian was one of Dr. Ann's finest managers, but he took the bold step of leaving her and striking out on his own 1,000 miles south in the sunshine state. Today, the "new" Hippocrates is a powerful beacon lighting the way for thousands to find healing through living foods and wheatgrass.

A visit to Hippocrates (HHI) requires a minimum of one week, but the recommended course is the three week *Life Change Program* designed to teach participants to take personal responsibility for health and recovery. Even though there are two medical doctors on staff (bring your medical records and drugs), this is not a medical facility. It is closer to a nutrition school/retreat than a hospital. You must be committed to working on yourself and be self-sufficient, or come with a personal assistant. The staff views themselves more as mentors than doctors. While hospitals may sicken you with their food and medicines and depress you with their manner and ambiance, HHI makes you come alive with its exquisite natural surroundings, positively motivated good company and therapies that are enjoyable rather than painful. They have three pools purified with ozone instead of chlorine, a whirlpool, a far-infrared sauna, and a cold plunge pool. Their exercise room is open 24 hours and has a variety of equipment including treadmills, rebounders, a vibrosaun, (a vibrating dry sauna) a hydrosonic bed, bio-rhythmic equalizer, and you can jog on the nature trail around the pond.

Their therapy building is located by a lake and includes colonic irrigation, massage, hydrotherapy, acupuncture, reflexology, homeopathy, chiropractic, kinesiology, psychotherapy, darkfield microscopy, yoga, shiatsu, deep-tissue massage, lymphatic drainage, hyperbaric chambers, aqua chi, several oxygen therapies, raindrop therapy, vitamin C drip, polarity energy balancing, and more. They also offer magnetic therapy in which you lie inside a magnetic field that increases the ion exchange between the inner and outer cell walls enhancing cellular function even in hard-to-reach places. While healing to the body, these therapies also relax the mind and enhance the spirit.

Hippocrates grows its wheatgrass in an air-conditioned greenhouse that has the magic touch of master grower, Michael Bergonzi, who renovated it in 2001. They have some of the best looking and best tasting greens in the U.S.–including wheatgrass, sunflower, pea greens, and buckwheat lettuce–all grown in soil. And you can get Bergonzi's *How to Grow Wheatgrass* DVD in their store. Their "self-service" wheatgrass bar is open 24 hours per day. Although it depends on your needs, expect to go on a juice fasting-detoxification program with colonics, enemas and wheatgrass implants. You will be able to juice fast as many days as you like because HHI offers three nutritionally balanced green drinks every day. When you're ready to eat solid food, it will all be life-giving foods. Expect to be delighted. If raw foods sound boring to you, your three weeks at Hippocrates will teach you how to prepare feasts that will nourish your cells in addition to pleasing your palate.

Hippocrates Buffet—Neither Cooked Nor Boring

Almond Basil Loaf with Red Pepper Coulis	Spelt Tortilla Rolls
Homey Hummus	Sliced Red Bell Peppers
Stuffed Avocado Platters	Dulse (Purple Sea Vegetable)
Cauliflower and Mushrooms a la Greque	Gorgeous Green Salad
Rose Sauerkraut	Sprout Medley
Sunflower Nori Sushi	Fresh Corn on the Cob

While here, you will dine on the finest organic veggies and sprouts available, plus watermelon juice (in season), organic herbal teas, lemon water and, of course, wheatgrass. There are several food preparation/ sprouting lectures, demos, and sampling throughout the three-week course.

Accommodations are some of the most exquisite available for a wheatgrass & living food retreat. They have a wide range of apartments and guest houses both on and off premises. Most have a stucco, terra-cotta theme. All of the off premise facilities are within walking distance. Some rooms include private baths, others have sunken tubs and jacuzzi's. Even the most economical rooms are perfectly comfortable.

Hippocrates also offers a *Health Educator Course* that is an intensive, nine-week training program for those who want to incorporate some of the lifestyle, nutritional and therapeutic disciplines practiced at Hippocrates in their profession. A fair number of people actually change careers and start growing wheatgrass and sprouts or become nutritional counselors or pursue other alternative health professions. The Educator Course takes place three times each year, and includes all of your meals, green drinks, wheatgrass juices, lectures, and exercises, seven days a week. Visit their website for more details, rates, and dates.

After your stay, or even before, you can keep up with the Hippocrates program by becoming a member. Membership fees are very modest and they stay in touch with you through mailings and their informative quarterly magazine. Some topics featured in previous magazines are: Light–Medicine of the Future; What We Know Now About Food That We Didn't Know Then; Staying Flexible in Body and Mind; Relationship-Voyages Through Life; Self-Esteem-The Mirror of the Mind.

HHI offers open-house tours every Thursday and Saturday at noon. And there are periodic lectures for the general public on growing wheatgrass and preparing raw food meals from scratch. Check the calendar page on their website for dates. They also offer fun alumni trips once a year.

It's not only the nutrients and phytochemicals in wheatgrass that make it therapeutically viable, it's the oxygen and electrical properties of the fresh living juice.

—Brian Clement, director

Optimum Health Institute—San Diego
6970 Central Avenue, Lemon Grove, CA 91945-2198.
619-464-3346, Fax 619-589-4098, 800-993-4325.
www.Optimumhealth.org

Before this way of living began for me, I was well over 200 lbs., and survived on any pill, fast food, alcohol, or any other relief available. I was a captive in my own house and in my own body. I had five surgeries, all related to food and self-abuse. Today, I am a trim, vibrant, fifty year old woman, in love with life. I have friends who, including myself, would not be alive today if it were not for the Optimum Health Institute. —Katie

Next to Ann Wigmore's original (now gone) institute in Boston, this is the oldest wheatgrass retreat center in the world. After her stay with Dr. Ann in 1976, Raychel Solomon was inspired to establish a similar center on the west coast of the U.S. Raychel opened *Hippocrates West* in 1976 with Dr. Ann's blessing and the help of Robert and Pamela Nees.

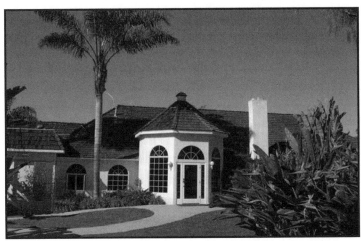

The entrance to Optimum Health Institute, San Diego

The name later changed to *Optimum Health Institute (OHI)* when they became part of the Free Sacred Trinity Church, which espouses Essene and Judeo/Christian teachings. This gives them non-profit status and enables them to minister mind, body, and spirit healing services at a very affordable price. Since then over one hundred thousand people have passed through their doors, and all of them have experienced the benefits of wheatgrass. A maximum of 155 guests can stay here at one time making it the largest wheatgrass training center in the world. Not only that but it's full most of the year and they all come by word of mouth—no advertising. There is a feeling of community here, alumni often come back for 'tune-ups.' The staff is so loyal, some came as guests decades ago and never left.

Being relatively close to Hollywood, this center has had many celebrities walk through its doors. Ben Vereen, the Beach Boys, Mrs. Sammy Davis, Jr., Edie Adams (wife of Ernie Kovacs), Lane Smith, Debbie Reynolds, Joel Douglas (son of Kirk) and Ernie Banks of the Chicago Cubs are just some who discovered wheatgrass at OHI.

The philosophy and methods of this institute are very close to those of Dr. Ann. They believe that, given the chance, the human body is self-regenerating and self-cleansing and that to improve the physical body, you must also work on the mental and spiritual. Balance and harmony are the goals and detoxification, wheatgrass, and living foods are the means.

Classes

Although you can stay more or less, the basic recommended program here is three weeks. It takes that long for the body to begin the detoxification process and for the person to learn the entire program well enough to take it home. The first week's classes are primarily theoretical in nature—how the body, mind, and spirit work together to create "dis-ease," or health. In the second week, classes are more practical, such as demonstrations on how to make fermented foods and on growing wheatgrass and sprouts. During the third week, students prepare and serve the living foods buffet to the second weekers, giving them actual hands-on experience before they go home.

Three Weeks to Rejuvenation

First Week	Second Week	Third Week
Daily Exercise	Daily Exercise	Daily Exercise
Mental Detoxification	Sprouting Instruction	Hands-on food preparation
Elimination	Mental Detoxification II	Sauerkraut making
Fasting	Fermented Foods	Dehydrating Foods
Emotional Detoxification	Emotional Detoxification II	Seed Sauces
Digestion	Wheatgrass Planting	Mind-Body Connection
Instant Relaxation	Organic Gardening	Transition Diet
Know Your Body	Communication	Equipment
Food Combining	Personal Care	Self-Esteem
Wheatgrass Instruction	Menu Planning	At-Home Follow-Up

Therapies and Food

This institute sticks to the basics. OHI operates on the principle that the body heals itself if given the proper tools. Their program of detoxification and raw foods is designed for self-healing and rebalancing. Raw juices, enemas, and wheatgrass implants are the essential therapies here. They believe that through detoxification and proper nourishment, the entire body, mind, and spirit becomes rejuvenated—which is the restoration of normal health.

Services such as massage, chiropractic, and colon hydrotherapy are available on the campus, but run as independent businesses and paid for separately. The exercise room is low impact and focuses mostly on cleansing the lymph system via rebounding on a trampoline.

The diet follows strict food combining principles and is all raw. Fermented foods such as rejuvelac, sauerkraut, and seed sauces play an important role in the diet—aiding digestion, elimination, and colon health. Buckwheat and sunflower sprouts, greens, fruits, and fresh vegetables are available seven days per week. A juice fasting liquid diet is recommended during the first few days.

The Wheatgrass Cathedral

The stature this greenhouse holds at OHI is reflective of the importance of grass to their healing program. It is a fully automated state of the art building. This temple of green, houses 1,500 trays and harvests 130 new ones each day, making it one of the largest wheatgrass greenhouses in the world. As you enter the greenhouse, you can feel the power of these amazing greens. Thousands of trays of young wheatgrass, buckwheat lettuce, and sunflower greens call out to you. The sun is their only light source and the temperature is controlled by shades and circulating air. The science of growing wheatgrass indoors has been refined down to the most minute details—from organic seed, to rich composted soil, even to the speakers that serenade the grass with classical music.

Accommodations

The grounds are lovingly cared for at OHI with beautiful lawns, flowers, trees, an organic vegetable garden, and private places to meditate and pray. The accommodations are simple and functional, minus the finery and trappings of expensive vacation spas. OHI focuses on the inner-life, not the outer one. They have several suites and townhouses in addition to single and shared rooms. Prices are most affordable.

Medicines

This is not a medical facility. There are no doctors on staff. OHI does not treat disease. Instead they will help you marshal the physical, mental, emotional, and spiritual resources that enable natural healing. You must be able to take care of yourself, attend classes and be open minded to learning new ways of living and eating. Patients undergoing chemotherapy should not attend. Whereas chemotherapy compromises the immune system, wheatgrass and the other therapies used at OHI strengthen it. You can do the program before chemotherapy to strengthen your system or after to rid your body of chemotherapy's toxic effects. As far as continuing with your prescription drugs, you must make your own decisions.

Nutritional supplements are not encouraged because they impose upon the body's natural chemistry. Wheatgrass, on the other hand adapts to the body's needs in addition to providing a broad spectrum of over 80 different nutrients. This program is a truly holistic one, addressing all aspects of a person's health—mental, emotional and physical.

> *We don't address the illness per se. The human body is the greatest doctor on earth. We remove the roadblocks and the body starts healing itself. Then, you name it—AIDS, cancer, arthritis, there are no limits.* —Robert Nees, former director

Optimum Health Institute—Austin

800-993-4325, 512-303-4817, Fax 512-332-0106.
265 Cedar Lane, Cedar Creek, TX 78612
Reservations.Austin@Optimumhealth.org
www.Optimumhealth.org

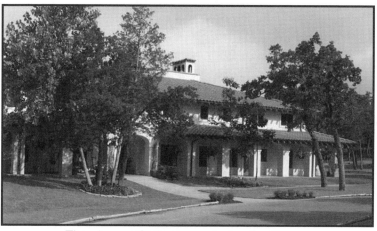

The elegant OHI campus in Austin, Texas.

As you place your feet on the massive stone floor entry, you begin to experience the quality and grandeur of the *Optimum Health Institute (OHI)* near Austin, Texas. Exquisite, yet rustic elegance is evident everywhere, from the custom built furniture, to the atrium court, to the grand oak stairway. The whole place is a labor of love.

Nestled in a park-like setting on 14 beautiful acres, the center is less than 20 minutes from Austin's new airport, offering both convenient

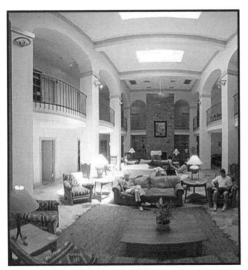

The lobby at OHI Austin.

access and country charm. Despite its proximity to a metropolitan area, there is a sense of peace and privacy here. A spiritual atmosphere is evident as you drive onto the beautiful grounds through a winding entry that reveals a large exquisite stucco and tile building. Its mission style architecture, textures and earthy colors add to the overall feeling of relaxed opulence.

This place was designed and built to be a health center and OHI was fortunate enough to acquire it. There is an exercise room with state-of-the-art equipment that overlooks the swimming pool and spa. The 20,000 square foot mansion houses 30 beautifully furnished bedrooms with all the amenities. It's obvious that quality standards for furniture, fixtures and equipment have not been compromised. There are also two distinctive suites that are just beyond a graceful and inviting walking path.

Austin OHI is managed by the same family as San Diego OHI and is also a not-for-profit church mission. It has the same philosophy and program as San Diego and tuition is comparable. (See San Diego for program information.) Both emphasize the holistic approach of physical, mental, spiritual, and emotional health, along with detoxification and wheatgrass. Both use independent practitioners for colon hydrotherapy, chiropractic, and massage. But the atmosphere in Texas is arguably more elegant and intimate.

The UK Centre for Living Foods

Holmleigh, Gravel Hill, Ludlow, Shropshire SY8 1Q. England
+44(0)1584-875308. Fax 015-887-5778. www.livingfoods.co.uk

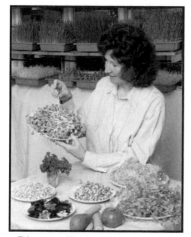

Director Elaine Bruce in the living foods kitchen at the UK Centre for Living Foods

I now think this was the best investment I have ever made in my health. My health and well being were dramatically improved during the course, but more importantly, the knowledge gained has empowered me to take total responsibility for my own health. Since this course in 1998 I have changed my career to Natural Healing and am now able to share this important knowledge with others.

—Sandra Hillawi

As soon as you enter the town of Ludlow, in the county of Shropshire, England, you know you are in a magical place. Here you will find rolling hills, gardens, castles, inns, cottages, farmhouses, forests, and old fashioned hospitality. Its timeless landscapes have inspired artists and writers for centuries. The town of Ludlow, where the institute is located, is itself a little gem. Although you are going to study, you never escape these magnificent surroundings.

The center is run by Elaine Bruce, who originally trained with Dr. Ann Wigmore in Boston in 1980. She has been practicing and teaching the Living Foods Program ever since. She served with the Ann Wigmore Foundation in Puerto Rico, and is also trained in Naturopathy and Homeopathy.

She started teaching the living foods lifestyle in the UK in 1990 and is the author of *Living Foods for Radiant Health*, and the video *A Teach-in with Elaine Bruce*.

The living foods courses are a blend of theory, discussion, and interactive hands-on work in the kitchen. A two-week stay is encouraged. The first week is busy with classes and theory. Then you'll roll up your sleeves and learn how to set up a living foods kitchen including juicing, composting, and growing wheatgrass and sprouts. The next week is devoted to detoxification. You'll learn about colon cleansing, fasting, wheatgrass enemas, and implants. The classes are small enough that Elaine can work with individuals to help plan their long-term diet and therapy program. In addition, there is a certified practitioner-training course to health professionals (and non-professionals) who wish to incorporate the Wigmore Living Foods Lifestyle methods into their practice.

You don't have to stay at the institute, but if you do, you will find the bedrooms pleasant, spacious, and clean. The shower room may include such amenities as a slant board and an elevated foot rest for la toilette. Then there is the beautiful garden sitting area, where one can enjoy the fresh air and the mild Shropshire weather. You'll also appreciate the organic permaculture garden, the compost and recycling area, and the store filled with living foods equipment and books. The menus include a variety of fresh local produce, garden herbs, juices, nut, and seed milks, patés, and sprouts. All in all, this center provides a rigorous education in a pastoral environment, with a friendly and supportive atmosphere.

Ann Wigmore Institute—Puerto Rico

PO Box 429, Rincon, Puerto Rico 00677. USA. 787-868-6307, fax 787-868-2430. www.AnnWigmore.org

On living foods, I completely healed from severe, inoperable cancer in my uterus, breast, and liver. Now I feel younger and better than ever. I feel I owe my life to the grace of God and Dr. Ann. —Mildred Rivera

Imagine the sound of the surf crashing on the beach and yoga by the sea. This is a refuge of beauty and tranquility where there is a natural propensity for inner purity that inspires an equilibrium with the pristine surroundings. This haven for purification of body, mind and spirit was one of the many gifts Ann Wigmore left us. Today, her spirit is still palpable in the cool breeze and her teachings are carried on faithfully by her devoted directors Leola Brooks and Lalita Salas.

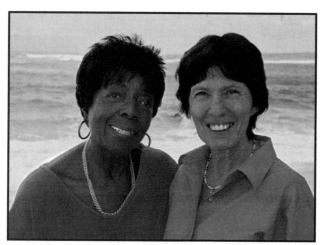

Leola Brooks and Lalita Salas. Two shining stars of
the living foods movement faithfully carry on Ann
Wigmore's teachings at her institute in Puerto Rico.

This institute was personally established by Dr. Ann and is among a
select few that teach her *Living Food Lifestyle*™ program in its original,
unmodified form. The flagship program is two weeks, but one week in-
tensives and one month discounts are also offered. Or, you can also just
go for a week of personal healing, which is less intensive. Much of the
course information described here applies to other centers listed in this
chapter, who teach the Living Foods Lifestyle program. The premise is
that natural, uncooked, and unprocessed food provides all of the living
enzymes, vitamins, minerals, proteins and amino acids necessary to nourish, protect, and defend the body's internal and external well-being.
When the body is cleansed and nourished, the symptoms of disease dis-
appear. Students learn about eating and cleansing and how to become
self-sufficient in growing and maintaining a lifestyle that encourages positive, physical, emotional, and spiritual well being.

Accommodations here range from private apartments, to private,
semi-private, and dormitory rooms. Prices are by the month or the week
and include the program, transportation to and from Mayaguez or
Aguadilla airports and meals. There are three simple, nurturing living
foods meals each day that include sprouted organic sunflower and buckwheat greens, alfalfa and other grain and legume sprouts, organic garden
grown veggies, fermented nut and seed yoghurts, veggie loafs, foods prepared in the dehydrator rather than the oven, energy soup, and rejuvelac.

The Ann Wigmore Living Foods Curriculum

Live food preparation	Dehydrating foods	Yoga and gentle exercise
Wheatgrass growing	Energy soup	Breathing and relaxation
Indoor gardening	Composting	Lymphatic exercises
Sprouting	Iridology and reflexology	Skin brushing and care
Enzyme nutrition	Detoxification	Lifestyle adjustment
Digestive health	Internal cleansing	Positive thinking
Rejuvelac	Colon health and hygiene	Meditation & visualization
Fermented foods	Enemas and Implants	Self-Esteem

Rejuvelac, energy soup, and wheatgrass are the cornerstone foods of Dr. Ann's Living Foods diet. Rejuvelac is a mildly fermented drink made from two to three day old wheat sprouts. It is the "fine wine" of living foods because it is aged into a rich brew of active enzymes and friendly bacteria. These *pro*biotics are more effective than *anti*biotics in fighting disease. Instead of killing bacterial invaders with antibiotics, probiotics compete against them until their numbers diminish and their threat is quashed. If there are more cops than burglars, the neighborhood is safe. Rejuvelac delivers lactobacillus, acidophilus, bifidus, and many other "friendly bacteria." They help control the intestinal environment against invading microbes, yeast, fungi, and parasites. These friendly bacteria also synthesize important B-vitamins. It's germ warfare in there and rejuvelac is your best armament. Yes, this is the same kind of protection you get from yoghurt, but rejuvelac is easier to digest, much more concentrated, and more economical in the volumes required to accomplish a change of inner terrain.

Energy soup is a thick shake or cold soup of super nutritious foods that are also easy to digest. Every food requires energy to digest. The ratio of energy received vs. energy spent on digestion determines how much net energy you will profit. If you fall asleep after eating a big meal of meat and potatoes, you have spent more than you earned. No matter how nutritious the meat is, you've lost. If this was the stock market, you would consider it a bad investment. Energy soup is like a golden parachute—your energetic profits are long lasting. The ingredients? It's a blended salad/soup of dulse, sprouts, indoor sunflower and buckwheat greens, organic garden greens, apple or papaya, avocado or almond cream and rejuvelac. There are many versions.

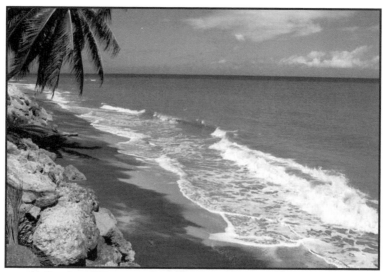

At the Ann Wigmore Institute in Puerto Rico, rejuvenation comes from living foods and also the ocean.

On a typical day, you may wake up to the birds singing, walk down to the beach for yoga, and afterwards make your own wheatgrass juice. Breakfast will be watermelon, papaya, or a fruit smoothie. Then it's off to classes. Lunch is energy soup, almond paté, and a buckwheat and sunflower sprout salad. Then it's back to classes to learn about colon care, enemas, and how to give yourself an implant. After a light dinner, there is time for a nice walk on the beach to enjoy the beautiful sunset. If there is a class in the evening, it will be something easy such as relaxation technique. Fourteen days of this and when you return home, your friends will take one look at you and ask: "Where have you been!"

The Ann Wigmore Foundation

PO Box 399, San Fidel, NM 87049.
505-552-0595, Fax 505-552-0595.
www.wigmore.org   Email: livingfood@wigmore.org

Dr. Ann founded the Hippocrates Health Institute in Boston in 1969 and later changed its name to the Ann Wigmore Foundation. She also started the Ann Wigmore Institute in Puerto Rico. Since the Boston fire in 1994, the original foundation has been closed *(see Epilogue)*. But now, the Ann Wigmore Foundation has been reborn in the spiritual heartland of New Mexico, just one hour west of Albuquerque.

The main learning center is an adobe building with rooms for dining, kitchen, sauna, colonics, massage and a central common room. The other two buildings on the property are residences for guests and staff. These natural wood octagon structures provide for eight private and semi-private rooms and dormitories. There is room for over twenty students and you get plenty of personal attention from long-time living foods lifestyle director Susan Lavendar. The greenhouse is a geodesic dome structure that is heated in the winter by solar energy. The New Mexico climate is very temperate. Although it can be 95°F in the summer, the inside rooms are cool enough even without fans. Winters average 50–60°F most of the time. With its vegetable garden, solar energy, and the indoor sprout gardens, this institute abides by Dr. Ann's philosophy of self-sufficiency.

Here, the original, unrevised Ann Wigmore program can be found. The one to three week program emphasizes Dr. Ann's philosophy of restoring health through cleansing the body and renourishing it with living foods. Teaching is geared to a learn-by-doing style. Classes are about the growing, juicing, and preparing of easy-to-digest, live-enzyme foods along with colon cleansing techniques such as wheatgrass enemas and implants. You'll also learn sprouting, indoor gardening, nut and seed fermentation, blending, dehydrating and composting. The emphasis is on successfully getting you to a place where you can continue the diet and lifestyle after your return to the larger society.

Mainstream eaters would term this fare spartan, but in fact it is very creative and definitely delicious. First thing every day is wheatgrass juice. This is a followed by a blended drink. Afternoon and evening meals may include energy soup, organic salads, sprouts of all kinds, seed, nut, and veggie loaves, nori rolls, or homemade sauerkraut. The sauerkraut is actually veggie-kraut made from different fermented root vegetables. The fermented foods, which include rejuvelac and seed sauces, provide an army of friendly bacteria that reclaim your digestive tract from putrefaction, giardia, parasites and yeasts. (Rejuvelac is made from young wheat sprouts before they turn into grass.) One day a week guests are served a liquid diet, and even that is loaded with variety and taste. A liquid salad is just as delicious as a real salad, but it is several times more concentrated in flavor and nutrition because the vegetables are all juiced. There are hands-on recipe classes for making rejuvelac, seed sauces, veggie and nut loaf, energy soup, almond milk, almond cream, dairy-free ice cream, and flourless desserts. It is quite gourmet.

Exercise, yoga, meditation and massage are sprinkled throughout the program. As with most of the other institutes, there are no medical doctors here. Neither is there any diagnosis. There is only one treatment for everyone—cleansing and renourishing of the whole person—body, mind and spirit.

From the medical evidence and my years of experience in observing people with all kinds of problems, I am convinced that young grasses, alfalfa and other chlorophyll-rich plants are a safe and effective alternative treatment for ailments such as high blood pressure, obesity, diabetes, gastritis, ulcers, pancreas and liver problems, osteomyelitis, asthma, eczema, hemorrhoids, skin problems, fatigue, anemia, halitosis, body odor, and constipation. I have found chlorophyll to be effective in alleviating symptoms of oral infection, bleeding gums, burns, athlete's foot, and cancer. —Dr. Ann Wigmore[1]

Creative Health Institute

112 West Union City Road, Union City, MI 49094. USA.
866-426-1213, 517-278-6260, fax 517-278-5837.
www.CreativeHealthInstitute.us

Since 1976, Creative Health Institute has taught and practiced the Dr. Ann Wigmore Living Foods Lifestyle program. We bear witness to the reversal of a wide range of diseases, and we strongly agree with Dr. Ann's belief: "There are no incurable diseases, just people who won't make the effort to restore wellness." —Donald O. Haughey, Founder, CHI

Located in an unpretentious setting in the central U.S., *Creative Health Institute (CHI)* provides a simple home away from home where one can walk country roads, meditate alongside the quiet Coldwater River, relax, cleanse and rejuvenate. This institute follows the Ann Wigmore Living Foods Lifestyle™ program. Founder Donald O. Haughey was a student of Dr. Ann's in the 1970s and has remained faithful to her work ever since. He is motivated by the spirit of helping others.

CHI is not a spa, nor is it a clinic. It is a non-profit teaching facility providing a program of natural body purification, nutrition, and rejuvenation through the use of fresh raw fruits, vegetables, juices, nuts, sprouted seeds, grains, beans, chlorophyll-rich greens and wheatgrass juice. Director Darcy Flynn says: "We offer no cures, we do not treat or heal. We teach. We share the information developed by Dr. Ann Wigmore about how a raw living foods lifestyle can benefit everyone as a total health solution, and how the body often cures itself with a proper diet." CHI does not sell supplements nor remedies, they simply provide loving guidance and hands-on experience.

Creative Health Institute's two-week program focuses on physical, mental, emotional, and spiritual wholeness. You wake up, have a wheatgrass juice and start exercising. During the day you'll watch training videos covering topics on the Living Foods Lifestyle program (see *Ann Wigmore Foundation*) such as sprouting, indoor gardening, composting, raw food preparation, and colon health. Then you'll proceed into the kitchen or the sprouting room and start applying what you've learned. CHI teaches self-responsibility. You're on your own a lot of the time here, as you would be if you were home. But the difference here is there is staff to answer your questions and other students around for support and sharing. Occasionally, well known speakers in the raw foods world drop in for a visit to this quiet, unspoiled haven, so check the schedule for guest speakers. There is enough free time for you to take advantage of the a-la-carte services such as massage and colonics. And then there are the meals! They're big beautiful buffets serving the finest raw foods, from nut milks, to seed cheeses, dehydrated veggie treats, energy soup, enormous sprout salads, juices, and more. The meals are a training in themselves. Long ago, there was a strong Christian underpinning to this place because of Don Haughey's ministerial background. But today, all religions and spiritual paths are welcome here.

Living Foods Institute

1530 Dekalb Avenue, NE, Suite E, Atlanta, GA 30307. USA.
800-844-9876, 404-524-4488. www.LivingFoodsInstitute.com

When a person truly has faith and belief in healing, there
is no disease too difficult or impossible to heal.

—Brenda Cobb, director

This is just what is needed—a training center in a major metropolitan area with lots of services and a flexible schedule. Unlike the other centers in this chapter, the *Living Foods Institute (LFI)* of Atlanta does not provide rooms. Instead you can choose from a broad selection of nearby hotels, some with shuttle service. Often, when you are making decisions about theses centers, the accommodations are a limiting factor. Not here! You can pick from two star to five star rated hotels to suit your budget and your comfort level. And you'll be learning from the best. Director Brenda Cobb is herself a survivor of breast and cervical cancer. She refused conventional treatment and turned to living foods. She completely changed her lifestyle and diet, lost 72 pounds, looks younger, and is cancer-free. Now she is energized to teach.

LFI offers a ten day training course. In it you'll get lots of kitchen practice and classes on sprouting, nutrition, food combining, acid-alkaline balancing, fasting, detoxification, prayer, herbs, essential oils, and the role of emotions in disease. The sessions, which run from 9PM–6PM daily, include meals, a training manual, a colon cleansing kit, and a range of optional treatments such as colonics, reflexology, chi machine, Bach Flower remedies, and energy work. If you can't find ten days, you can stay for as long as you can and finish at a later time. Want to test it out first? No problem. Free seminars are offered every month to the general public. And if you just want to visit for a detox treatment, that's okay, too. For many, LFI is the best of both worlds. It's easy to get to, has a flexible schedule, a full line of services, and the education is topnotch.

Hippocrates Health Centre of Australia

Elaine Ave, Mudgeeraba 4213, Gold Coast,
Queensland, Australia.
Tel. (61)075-530-2860. www.hippocrates.com.au

I've lost a lot of weight in four weeks here. I've stopped smoking once and for all. My skin is clearer. My eyes are shiny again. Chronic fatigue is gone. I feel fully energized. I've gained an incredible amount of knowledge about my mind and body and I've developed the self-discipline necessary for me to continue to blossom at home. —Jennifer Blake, Hornsby, NSW

The Hippocrates Health Centre of Australia was started in 1985 with the blessings of Dr. Ann Wigmore. Ronald Bradley is a faithful adherent to the principles set forth by Dr. Ann. She gave him the use of the Hippocrates name and logo—something that she did not part with easily. Here you will find the unblemished version of Dr. Ann's teachings in all its simplicity and wisdom.

The recommended program here is three weeks. But you can go for less or stay for more. Experience has shown that the longer you stay, the better your success in maintaining the diet/lifestyle after you return home. This institute closely follows the Ann Wigmore Living Foods Lifestyle program. (For details, see the *Ann Wigmore Institute* in this chapter.) Tuition fees include most everything you'll need including an iris analysis, private health assessment, and personal counseling. Massage, ear candling, saliva hormone testing, homeopathy, and other such services are extra.

If you ever wanted to visit Australia, this is a great excuse! And, because of currency exchange rates, it is still a bargain for North Americans and Europeans willing to fly over. That shortens the psychological distance of this otherwise far away and down under retreat. But be prepared to write a letter or make a phone call. Public faxing, web browsing, and e-mailing are not available at this low-tech location. You'll have to phone or write a letter to make inquiries and arrangements. Check your clock before you call. They are 14 hours ahead of New York time. The accommodations are private motel-style suites that hold a maximum of fourteen people when full. Privacy and personal care here are at the highest level.

Grow Your Own

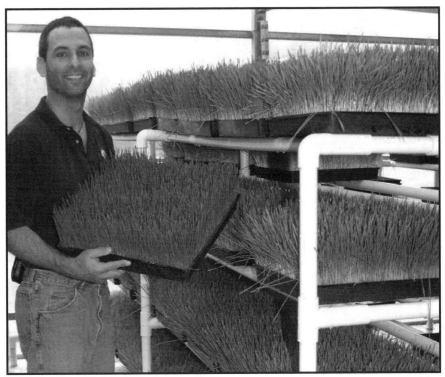

Master Grower Michael Bergonzi in the Hippocrates Greenhouse

This chapter is about wheatgrass, not wheat grass. As explained in the primer at the beginning of this book, "wheat grass" is grown outdoors in the field and "wheatgrass" is the term applied to the therapeutic use of the indoor grown grass. You can learn about the many differences between these two grasses in the chapter on *Healing*. Since most of you are not farmers, indoor gardening is the most practical way to grow your own grass. This chapter tells you how to do it. There are many pitfalls to growing your own grass. But you're in the right place. These pages are full of garden wisdom. You'll learn about soil and non-soil methods, find troubleshooting tips, get growing advice from experts, comparisons of costs, and even learn how to make your own hydroponic grower. So roll up your sleeves. It's time to get down and dirty.

How to Grow Wheatgrass in Soil

Seeds & Trays. Purchase organic hard wheat berries, either winter or spring wheat, from a natural food store, a mail order sprouting seed supplier or your local wheatgrass grower (see *Resources*). If buying from a store, try to find packaged seed as opposed to bulk bin seed that has suffered from exposure to air and moisture. There is nothing else in the growing process that is more critical than the selection of seed. More on this later. Purchase "seeding trays" from any garden store. Some common sizes are 11 by 11 or 11 by 21 inches. Buy the kind without holes in the bottom, since you don't want a leaking tray. If the retailer doesn't have your size, they can order it.

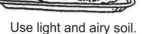

Use light and airy soil.

Soil. The best soil is light and airy with an approximate mix of 50% peat moss, 40% organic top soil, and 10% vermiculite, pearlite or other aerators. This is considered a "deluxe potting soil" formula commonly available at garden stores. Anything close to this formula will do.

Sprout Bag Seed Starter. A sprouter is needed to pre-germinate your seeds before planting. Sprouting bags are preferred over jars. As the inventor of the flax and later the hemp sprouting bag, this author is completely biased in favor of bags over jars. But that is only because they work a thousand times better! For starters, bags never break and never mold. Unlike jars, they breathe and drain perfectly and involve less handling—just dip and hang. They save space too. They can hang out on a cup hook or cabinet knob, or lay in a dish rack or bowl. Jars have held a curse over sprouting for decades. They retain water and suffocate the sprouts with insufficient air circulation—perfect conditions for growing mold. How they became synonymous with sprouting is one of those cultural mysteries along the lines of "milk builds strong bones" and "white bread builds muscles." No one ever designed jars to be gardening tools. Nevertheless, you can certainly use them, if you take good care. But if you are ready to enter the world of trouble-free sprouting, get hold of a few sprout bags. (See *Resources.*)

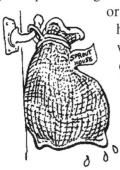

Sprout bags are the easiest way to get your seeds started.

Basic Steps for Growing Grass in Soil

1. Soak 2 cups of grain for 9–12 hours
2. Sprout for 2 days, rinsing twice per day
3. Lay seeds on top of soil
4. Water with a sprinkler head spout
5. Cover the seedlings
6. Set seedling tray in a shady spot
7. Check daily and moisten if necessary
8. Remove cover when 2–3 inches tall
9. Expose to light; water daily
10. Harvest in 10–14 days or 7–10 inches tall.

Ten Steps to Success

Step 1. Soak 2 cups of grain in a jar of pure water for 9–12 hours.

Step 2. Drain out the soak water and rinse the seeds well in fresh water. Germinate the seeds for two days in a sprout bag rinsing at least twice per day.

Step 3. Fill your seedling tray with 1–2 inches of soil.

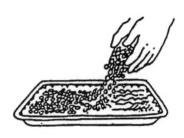

Lay the sprouted grain evenly on top of the soil one level deep.

Step 4. After 2 days of germinating in the sprouter, the seedlings are ready for planting. Healthy seedlings will have a single thick shaft emerging from the grain and several white hairlike rootlets. Lay the seedlings on top of the soil spreading them evenly. Two cups of dry grain nicely fills a standard 11 by 21 inch seedling tray. But if you are using a different size tray, simply lay out enough seeds to cover the surface one level deep.

Step 5. Water the entire tray with pure water using a watering can that has a sprinkler head. The sprinkler is important in order to get a gentle and even shower. Water only enough to moisten the soil. Be careful not to over water. There are no drainage holes in the tray. Excess water will fester and create mold.

Step 6. Cover the entire tray by laying a second tray on top. The cover tray can either be nested into the seedling tray or inverted and placed on top sandwich style. Heard about covering the tray with a plastic garbage bag or newspaper? Don't do it.

Water only to moisten the soil then cover with a second tray.

It fosters mold and leaches out newsprint chemicals. That is just another piece of misguided information. (We have enough of that, don't we!) The idea is simply to keep moisture in and light out. If using a bag, tuck it in loosely around the edges. It's not an air tight cover and it doesn't have to be.

Step 7. Set the tray in a shady spot away from extremes of cold, heat, or wind. Wheatgrass grows best in cool weather. The ideal temperature would be 70°F. (21°C), but it can vary.

Step 8. Check your crop daily–without fail–to make sure the seedlings are not drying out. Water only if they're dry. A mister or atomizer is ideal at this stage for adding a small amount of water to the seedlings without significantly wetting the soil. That's the secret!

Step 9. When the sprouts reach approximately 2 inches in height (about 3 days), start watering with your watering can. Water once daily, being careful to use only enough water to moisten the soil. Tip: If you were to squeeze the soil in your hands, it would feel wet but not drip.

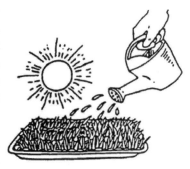

At the two inch height, the inverted cover lies loosely over the sprouts. At three inches, eliminate use of the cover and expose the growing grass to normal light.

When 3" tall, expose to light, and water daily.

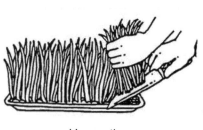

Harvesting

Step 10. Wheatgrass is mature and ready for harvest when 7–10 inches tall. This usually falls between 10 and 14 days depending on the climate. Another marker is when the blade develops a second stem. Harvest by cutting about one inch above the soil using a serrated knife.

The Troubleshooting Check List

1. Soil: lightweight and airy
2. Seed: test, test, and test
3. Watering: moist but not wet
4. Air: breeze or fan.
5. Temperature: aim for 70°F
6. Humidity: keep it low
7. Light: indirect light or shade or...
8. Direct sun—max. 3 hrs./day
9. Location, location, location
10. Season—too hot? too cold?

Troubleshooting Solutions
Tips to Make you a Gifted Gardener

About Soil

Quality of soil is critical. Most pre-mixed potting soils available at garden center stores are satisfactory. Deluxe potting soils usually include larger amounts of peat moss and soil aerators like vermiculite and perlite. Light and airy soil works best. You can make your own soil from organic compost. Dr. Ann Wigmore is famous for having designed a method of composting indoors in a bucket with worms yet having no smell! Compost increases the nutritive value of the soil and thus your grass. You can start two growing trays side by side from the exact same seed, same growing conditions and the grass with composted soil will be taller, greener, fatter, and juicier. The secret is in the compost. If you are interested in composting, pick up a good book on the subject. Although the subtleties of composting can get quite technical, the process is fairly simple. After all, the worms do most of the work!

Seed Quality and Storage

Seed quality should be your highest priority. The seed you choose may very well make the difference between an easy-to-grow, trouble-free crop and a harvest of mold and headaches. "Organic" is not good enough. It merely defines a method of agriculture. It does not guarantee you gorgeous grass. Not at all. Good grass-growing grain is generally low in moisture and high in protein. That means under 10 percent for moisture and about 12 percent or better for protein. Nevertheless, these numbers do not tell the whole story. The only way to really know for sure is to test. Order small quantities from different suppliers and start testing. Or, call the local wheatgrass grower and either buy seed from him or get his recommendation. Good seed is golden.

Grass can be grown successfully from hard winter or hard spring wheat. Soft wheat is not recommended. Kamut®, the ancient Egyptian, non-hybrid Durham type wheat, makes an excellent grass. The grain is generally 17–18 percent protein and makes mild tasting, thick grass blades. *Green Kamut Corporation* is a company that grows grass from this type of wheat in the high plains of Utah (see *The Companies*). Barley is a wonderful seed for growing grass and many claim that it is nutritionally superior to wheat. *Green Magma* is the most popular barley grass juice powder with volumes of scientific research behind it. The seed however, is not available at any natural food stores and cannot be special ordered from them. Your only luck will be through the specialty seed mail order suppliers

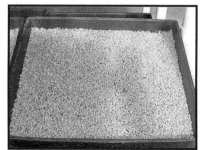

Two day old sprouted wheat laid evenly, one layer deep, on top of soil.

Photo by R. Ross, Optimum Health Inst.

(see *Resources*) who carry un-husked barley for the specific purpose of sprouting. Don't even think about testing the barley sold in health stores. Once you've got the right seed, you'll enjoy this slightly taller and broader blade. Oats are even harder to obtain than barley. Although animal feed stores will provide both, the high amount of debris in their product makes them unsuitable for sprouting. Rye and spelt are available in many natural food stores and are similar to wheatgrass.

You may need to buy seed in volume, especially if you discover a good batch. Here's how: Store your grain in a cool dry place. Basements are usually good for coolness but bad for moisture. A perfectly sealed storage bucket (with a moisture proof lid) is the only way to prevent moisture and vermin damage. Don't buy bulk seed in the spring or summer. Grain is difficult to store in hot weather. Buy it in the fall when you will have nine months of winter temperatures for cool storage.

Setting Up Your Growing Room

Your growing location should have convenient access to water, light and working space. If necessary, you can choose to use indoor grow lights and a watering can. Shelves can be located on the window, on the wall or as a stand alone unit. Shelf brackets and shelves are readily available at hardware stores and are easy to install. Space the two vertical brackets so

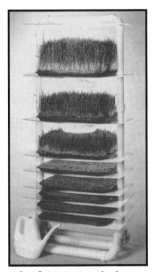

An 8 tray stand-alone grower from Sundance Industries.

that each shelf is divided into three sections for three trays. Since each pair of brackets can support 3–4 horizontal shelves, this enables a 9–12 tray capacity. Stand alone units can also be constructed with four legs and can be 6 feet high fitting 16 trays. Visit your garden center store or put on your tool belt and build it yourself.

Light

Little or no light is required during the first four days of germination. Dark or shady areas are best. That is why the seedlings are covered with a second tray. After this time, place your sprouter in indirect sunlight, i.e. room light or a bright area. Avoid direct sunlight immediately after uncovering. Sun is both good and bad, just as with people. Sunlight on the soil keeps mold in check, but without proper ventilation can raise temperatures to 100 degrees (38°C) and cook your grass. Just one exposure of this heat is enough to start the process of rot, bacterial growth, and mold.

The first five days of growth are critical.
This is the time when most growing problems originate.

If your location exposes your grass to several hours of direct sun, you will need to increase its diet of water. The more light, the faster and taller they will grow, but also the faster they will dry out. So monitor them carefully. Indirect sun provides more balanced temperatures and even growing conditions. Since there are fewer highs and lows in temperature and moisture, there are fewer problems.

Open a window to circulate the air or use a slow fan. If there are long periods of direct sun without a breeze, the grass may overheat. Relocate your crop to a shady spot if necessary. Three hours of sunlight per day is plenty. If you do not have sunlight, grass can grow its entire life in indirect light, shade or with full spectrum grow lights.

Harvesting

Harvest time is going to be slightly different for every location. The general recommendation is 10–14 days. Look at your grass. If it is starting to lean over, or is turning yellow, it will not be very nutritious. Better to

cut the grass and refrigerate it while
it still looks good than have it go ge-
riatric on you. The inch or two of soil
limits how long the grass can live. But
there is no law limiting you to growing in two inch tall trays. If you grow
your grass in a terra-cotta planter with
10 inches of soil, you can achieve
greater longevity, better nutrition,
and milder taste.

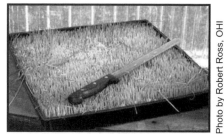

Freshly harvested! Yum!

Photo by Robert Ross, OHI

Pure Water

Water is your primary ingredient. It is the river on which all life flows.
If this grass is your medicine, you surely want to use the highest quality
water. Purchasing bottled water is uneconomical because of the volumes
involved. You should be drinking, cooking, sprouting and washing vegetables in pure water, so a home water purifier is the best choice. Distilled
water, loose granular carbon filters, hard carbon block filters and reverse
osmosis are your options. Since plants thrive on mineral content, you can
add liquid kelp, *Ocean Grown,* rock dust, or another source of minerals to
any of these waters to enrich them. This is especially valuable for hydroponic
gardening and anytime you use distilled water since it is mineral-free.

Nagging Gnats

These tiny fruit flies show up for dinner whenever mold is present because that's what they eat! They won't hurt the grass, but they will annoy
you. Your best solution is to grow mold-free wheatgrass. But if you are
stuck with them, here are a few tips. Get an exhaust fan and sit the grass
tray in front of it. Hang up fly paper. Keep your vacuum armed and ready.

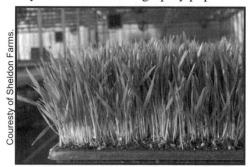

Couresty of Sheldon Farms.

It's war! If you have a bad infestation, wash and clean your entire growing area. Sanitize. If it
is wintertime, chill the growing
room for a good few hours.
That will give you a fresh start.
Before you resume operation,
carefully follow the steps on
how to grow mold-free grass.

Mature wheatgrass ready to harvest.

How to Store Your Fresh Cut Grass

Sprout bags, glass, plastic containers with lids, or green eco-storage bags are the best way to extend the life of your refrigerated grass. Standard plastic bags are not recommended. They suffocate grasses and vegetables, too. Sprout bags are natural hemp fiber sacks that breathe and drain perfectly. Unlike plastic bags, they won't create puddles of water that breed bacteria and mildew. A plastic or glass container is also good because it allows air circulation and has some airspace at the top. Green *Evert-Fresh* storage bags are chemically different from standard plastic bags and measurably increase the longevity of your refrigerated crop. Good grass cut in its prime and refrigerated in this manner can last over two weeks.

Don't eat yellow-tinged grass. Juice your grass before it starts to turn. If you have more grass than you can use, juice it and pour it into ice cube trays. One day when you are out of grass, you can drop a grass ice cube into a carrot juice and you will still benefit from it.

Coping with Mean Mister Mold

Molds, fungi, and other microorganisms are a part of gardening—especially organic gardening where no chemical fungicides, insecticides, or mold inhibitors are used. Mold is the bane of all wheatgrass growers. It is unsightly, unappetizing, it ruins crops, and also, as it turns out, is quite controversial.

Does Mold Cause Nausea?

Just like hanging chads on voting ballots, steroids in sports, and cilantro in your salad, wheatgrass has achieved enough notoriety to become controversial. It's true! Some people can get a little nauseous when drinking wheatgrass juice—on this all concur. The controversy surrounds the question: "why?" Some allege that it is the mold growing on tray-grown wheatgrass that causes nausea and other allergic responses. The other camp claims the mold is harmless. They argue that any intense drink can cause nausea in some people. Drinking too much garlic juice, for example, will also upset the stomach. There are truths on both sides. So, let's take a closer look.

Carroll J. MacIntosh, of *Evergreen Wheatgrass* growers in Canada, used to grow wheatgrass indoors until she decided she could not serve it anymore—"knowing that all the so called detox symptoms were reactions to the mold." She says: "Mold is highly toxic and can cause instant reactions such as headaches and nausea and even hives." Evergreen grows its grass outdoors where the wind and sun prevent mold development.

Carroll is right. Tray-grown wheatgrass is prone to mold development. But is this mold the cause of nausea and headaches? Or is it something else? If you decide to grow your own wheatgrass, are you doomed to also grow mold? Here are a few things to consider.

How to Avoid Nausea

Drinking something as intense as wheatgrass juice on a partially full stomach will definitely clash with the leftovers in the stomach. Drink wheatgrass juice on an empty stomach or not at all. Wheatgrass juice requires some adaptation. If you are new to this juice, start with one ounce per day and slowly build up until you can tolerate more. Even experienced fresh wheatgrass drinkers can only tolerate about four ounces at a time. Drinking six or eight ounces at one sitting is bound to upset even the strongest stomach even if it is perfectly mold-free. But Carroll's remarks correctly point to another problem. Home wheatgrass growers have been known to grow some pretty bad grass—grass with mold, brown roots, and yellow blades. Drink-ing some of this substandard grass will most definitely sour your stomach or stimulate allergic reactions if you are sensitive in that way. It is the equivalent of drink-ing sour milk—don't do it or you will pay the price.

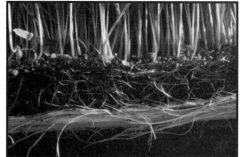

Perfect mold-free wheatgrass grown by Sheldon Farms. (This grass will soon get freeze-dried.)

Here is the big picture. Some people grow moldy wheatgrass; some are sensitive to mold, while others are not. Some folks simply drink more than they can tolerate and their stomachs rebel. There are a variety of nausea related issues converging at once, but there is hope. You are not doomed to grow mold with your wheatgrass. Read on.

The Four Types of Mold

There are actually four different kinds of mold on wheatgrass.

A) The most common type of mold is a white or gray cotton-like mold that forms a web of filaments around the seeds and lower ends of the stalks. This is most probably *rhizopus sp.* If caught early, it can be rinsed off. If it matures, you may notice some black spots. It is related to bread mold and is generally considered harmless in small quantities, but has the potential to cause problems for the elderly, children, or allergic people.

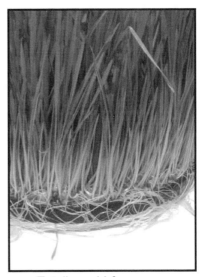

B) Also common is a mold that forms on the seeds themselves. It also could be *rhizopus*. It may be blue or gray or fuzzy and usually shows up around the fifth day. Wheatgrass is typically cut about an inch above the seeds so you should be safe—just rinse off the blades before juicing.

C) Root rot or brown roots are harmful to the plant. They spread like an infection up the stalk into the blades.

Totally mold-free grass grown without soil.

This is most likely *Pythium sp.* It is caused by too much moisture and not enough air. Don't harvest a crop with brown roots. It indicates that the plant is under attack and unhealthy plants should not be consumed. Be sure to sterilize your growing trays during cleanup so you do not transfer the spores to future crops grown in the same tray.

D) The last type of "mold" is not mold at all. It is the cilia hairs forming a fringe on the rootlets. As drops of moisture cling to them, they look very cottony. It shows up over the first few days and disappears with watering. If it keeps coming back, then it really is mold. The cilia hairs are reaching out for water. Take this as an indication that you are not watering enough.

Tips for Mold Free Wheatgrass

A) *Seed Quality.* The number one cause of mold on wheatgrass is bad seed. Yes, it must be hard wheat, not soft or white wheat. But it does not matter whether it is hard red winter or hard spring wheat. The problem is that wheatberries sold in stores are intended for bread baking. But the seed characteristics for good grass and good bread are completely different. The only way to determine quality is to test. Either you do the testing or you buy seed from a reputable sprouting and wheatgrass seed company who did the testing. Professional wheatgrass growers will test dozens of seeds before they select the perfect one. Buying from bulk bins in health food stores presents another problem. They sit there for weeks wicking up ambient moisture that degrades germination. Oh sure, you may get lucky. But if you want no-hassle wheatgrass with long dark green juicy blades and zero mold, buy from a wheatgrass and sprouting seed specialist (see *Resources*).

B) *Temperature*. Grass likes it cool. Grass is happiest around 70°F. (21°C) and unhappy around 90°F. (32°C). Heat promotes the development of spores and root rot.

C) *Air Circulation*. A fan in the growing room is very helpful to keep mold spores from ganging up.

D) *Soil*. Follow the soil suggestions in this chapter. Good airy soil eliminates many problems.

E) *Drainage*. Too much water stuck in the growing tray, or soil that is too wet, fosters the growth of mold.

The seed is the number one cause of wheatgrass mold.

Sometimes mold is a process of elimination—change the soil, change the trays, change the environment....but more often than any other factor, the problem is the choice of seed.

Mold Killers

Hydrogen peroxide is a natural, non-toxic mold killer. Spraying or misting the young seeds is helpful. Drug store hydrogen peroxide is readily available and cheap. Or you could buy the higher concentrated food-grade brand from specialty vendors (see *Resources*). Follow the dilution instructions on the bottle. Other products such as grapefruit seed extract also work. Even diluted bleach works, although it is not as environmentally preferable. All these products are helpful, but they are just band-aids. The best course of action is to eliminate the cause.

Zero Mold and other Growing Tips from Master Grower Michael Bergonzi

Michael Bergonzi has been the greenhouse manager for the two premier wheatgrass retreat centers in the world. He designed and built the state of the art greenhouse at the *Optimum Health Institute* in 1990 and at the time of this writing is the greenhouse manager of the *Hippocrates Health Institute* in Florida. (See *Resources.*) The author's questions are in italics.

How did you get started growing wheatgrass? In 1990, I got a job at the *Optimum Health Institute* in California. I had no plan to become a wheatgrass grower, but when the position opened up, I took it. When I first walked in the [greenhouse] door there was mold everywhere—on every tray of wheatgrass. Mold had to be my first priority. We were running out of grass for the guests. When I talk about mold, I mean mean the spider-web cotton-looking mold that grows up the grass. But you have to look closely. During the first few days of growth, the cotton you see may *not* be mold. It is actually the root hairs that are reaching for food [water]. When the grass is mature, there might also be a greenish type mold on the seeds. Do not be concerned, as we always harvest the grass above the seed. Also, you can still use the grass. Just rinse it off before juicing as this mold is "around" the grass.

What are your tips for controlling mold? First of all, there is no "quick fix" to get rid of the mold once it is on your grass. That said, here are four things I would recommend. First, *Control the Temperature.* Always keep it between 60–80°F. Secondly, *Create Air Circulation.* Blow air around the grass especially if the temps get above 80°F. Use a ceiling fan, an oscillating fan, an air conditioner, etc. Air movement will prevent 90 percent of all mold issues. I have grown mold-free wheatgrass successfully in 95°F. weather in Florida as well as 110°F. heat in northern California. *Plant Thin.* Use less seed per tray. This will allow more air to flow through your wheatgrass. *Change Your Seed.* If you have good air flow, and you are still getting mold, it is time to change the variety of wheat seed you are using.

Tell me more about the seed. Changing your seed source is what worked every time. Throughout the process of changing soil, temperature, watering, planting trays, air circulation, the things that worked the best for the spider-web, cotton-looking mold was *air movement,* and then changing the seed. There are over 1,500 varieties of wheat seed out there. I try to buy my seed from farmers that "summer sow" and put the nutrients back into the earth before planting their next crop of wheat. So, in turn, I get a seed with a better immune system. This makes all the difference. When all else fails, try a different wheat. I choose hard winter wheat, however there is a hard spring wheat that might be good, too. Soft wheat or white wheat will not work at all. Hard wheat is at times referred to as "wheatberries." However, they are seeds.

Can you recommend a strategy for fruit flys? Those pesky little flies show up when there is mold present. They are microorganisms that "hatch" when something starts to decompose. If you want to rid your wheatgrass of flies, increase your air circulation to get rid of the mold. Flies like warm air and no air flow. When they are in your home, use fly paper as well as a vacuum cleaner!

What about soil? I use a very basic potting mix or top soil from a bag. Organic soil, straight out of a bag, might cause more mold because it is acid based. Wheat likes a more alkaline soil.

What about growing without soil? Personally, I will always use soil for growing wheatgrass as well as sunflower greens, pea greens, and buckwheat lettuce rather than hydroponics. The reason for using soil is not for nutrition. It is something more than what science can prove at this point. It is for the "vibration-energy life-force" that you can see, feel, and taste in the greens. When Ann Wigmore healed herself from grass, it was grass grown in the earth. The message she learned was simple: Get the *Earth* back into our diets and more *oxygen* back in our blood.

Troubleshooting with Master Grower Richard Rommer

Richard Rommer grew wheatgrass for Dr. Ann Wigmore as early as 1973 while apprenticing at her *Hippocrates Health Institute* in Boston. His company, *Gourmet Greens,* is one of the few that ships fresh grass and soil-grown sprouts via refrigerated next day air in the USA. (See *Resources.*) The author's questions are in italics.

What's the most important thing you have to tell home growers? Sooner or later all wheatgrass growers encounter mold. It is a white or gray cotton looking growth at the soil level that if left unchecked will stunt the wheatgrass and even prevent the leaves from turning fully green. It is especially prevalent in the summer during hot humid days. There are several things the grower can do to keep mold to a minimum.

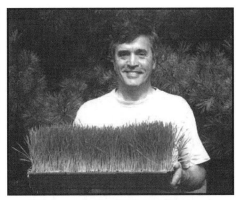

Master grower Richard Rommer

First, use good soil that is fully composted. Organic matter is great but if it is not fully broken down by beneficial microorganisms, it will contribute to the buildup of mold. If you are growing with a store-bought soil mix, make sure it is free of anything like bark or bits of hay or straw. It should be consistent and free flowing.

Second, get good seed. Many people start growing with a small bag of wheat purchased at a health food store and wonder why they can't grow good wheatgrass. That seed may be old or improperly stored and no one has tested it to see if it grows good wheatgrass. There is an abundant supply of good quality organically grown seed out there. Buy your seed from a wheatgrass grower or sprouting seed house that has tested it for their own use.

Any tricks on getting the seed started? Soak your wheatgrass seed in the refrigerator for 24 hours whenever you are having mold problems. This prevents the soak water from getting funky. And when you pour off the soak water, rinse it with plenty of clean water until all the colored soak water is gone. Let the seed sprout for about 12 hours before you spread it onto the trays.

We stack our trays with the bottom of one tray directly on top of the one beneath it for 48 hours at 67°F. At the end of the 48 hours, the trays are separated and transferred to the growing shelves.

What about water and light? Water immediately but do not overwater. Water only once a day. After one day, your trays should not be

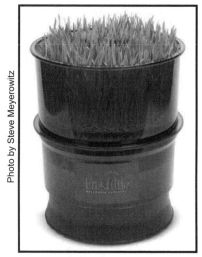

Grass grows happily–
and soil-free–in the
Freshlife Automatic Sprouter.

dried out—but they should need water. One half hour after watering, the soil should have the moisture of a wrung out sponge. That is, if you take the soil into your hand and squeeze gently no water should drip from your hand. But if you squeeze tightly, water will drip out.

If you live in a sunny climate, a greenhouse is best. Second best is good grow lights. The young shoots of the wheatgrass will follow the light. Good light getting down to the soil level will help to keep mold to a minimum. Harvest the grass before it begins to lose its vigor and fall over on its own. Once it falls over, you are no longer getting light down to the soil level.

A slow moving oscillating fan will keep the air moving. Direct the air flow directly onto the trays. This may tend to dry out the soil in the trays so keep an eye on the soil moisture. You want the young sprouts to have plenty of available water but they cannot be sitting in pools of water. Remember the wrung out sponge test.

Harvest the grass just before it starts to fall over. If it is more than you can use, store the extra wheatgrass in a plastic bag in the refrigerator at 34–37°F. Fresh harvested grass is best but don't think that yellowing, falling over grass is better than refrigerated wheatgrass. [*Fin*]

How to Grow Grass Without Soil

Traditionally, all grass—indoor or outdoor—has been grown in soil. All the major wheatgrass retreat centers grow it that way and Dr. Ann Wigmore, the mother of wheatgrass therapy, never endorsed any alternatives. That being said, can you grow grass successfully without soil? And is it as good?

Soil vs. Non-Soil

Robert Nees, former director of the largest wheatgrass retreat center in the world, *The Optimum Health Institute*, reported that once upon a time, they grew and served hydroponic (soil-free) wheatgrass to their guests. He said: "There is only a minor difference in nutrient value between the two grasses. We only stopped [growing hydroponic] because it was inefficient for us

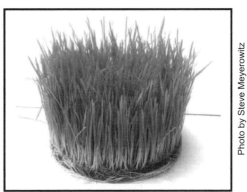

No mold. Wheatgrass grows nicely without soil.

Photo by Steve Meyerowitz

on a large scale." Dr. Chiu-Nan Lai, of the University of Texas System Cancer Center, used soil-free wheatgrass in her research and still reported that "the inhibition of activation of potent carcinogens is quite strong at a reasonably low level of extract." (See *Research*.)

Sure, soil is the natural medium for growing plants. But sprouts are traditionally grown without soil and wheatgrass is, after all, a kind of sprout. A sprout is a baby plant. You are basically eating the plant before it has a chance to develop a root system. If you compare the roots of the ten day old grass with the outdoor-grown sixty day old grass, you will notice a vast difference. The mature grass has a complex root system up to eighteen inches long. The ten day grass has slim two inch long roots. The immature roots of the young wheat are not yet capable of converting inorganic minerals into the organic form that they can uptake into the plant. The soil serves more as a structural support and a source for beneficial microorganisms. The hydroponic grass, on the other hand, can absorb lots of minerals by osmosis through the water. Enriching your water with sea minerals from liquid kelp or *Ocean Grown*, would be the best way of feeding the young plant.

Let's face it, growing grass in your home is easier if you don't have to use soil. There is simply less to do—less composting, less bugs, and less mold. Hydroponic grass also has a milder taste. Some people ask: "can you juice the whole grass, roots and all?" You can, but it is not a good idea. If there is any mold growth, it is going to be there, at the seed base and roots. So just stick to juicing the tops as usual. Soil-grown grass is arguably still superior and the most dependable for fighting a serious health challenge. But once you get your hydroponic gardening skills up to speed, you will be hard pressed to distinguish between the two grasses. Take this simple advice: Choose the method that best suits your circumstances. Either way, you're going to be a winner.

Did you say Hydroponics?

Hydroponics is a term we are borrowing from the conventional world where hydroponic tomatoes and lettuces are grown in a sandy bed or a synthetic nutrient solution instead of soil. It is the term that defines alternatives to soil based gardening. We don't use any commercial growth enhancement products, only liquid seaweed. For the most part, our use of the term infers just seed and water.

Hydroponic Grass Growers

Like other sprouts, wheatgrass will grow without soil. But, because wheatgrass has a more fibrous root system than other sprouts, ordinary sprouting devices won't do. Once upon a time, only commercial sprouters costing several thousand dollars were available. Today, there are a few manufacturers offering affordable soil-free wheatgrass growers for the home user and some of them can grow multiple levels. That means you can rotate your crops and achieve a continuous grass supply. Check the *Resources* chapter to get information.

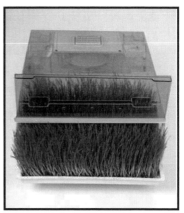

The EasyGreen hydroponic grass grower can grow up to 3 levels.

Build Your Own Grass Sprouter

Are you the do-it-yourself type? You can build your own hydroponic wheatgrass grower without much difficulty. The following are instructions on how to build a simple, soil-free grower. Keep in mind that most of the considerations about air circulation, light, temperature, water purity, etc. discussed earlier, also apply for soil-free gardening.

First pay a visit to your garden center store. There you will find lots of seed starters. You are going to use some of those materials for your non-soil adventure. Look for plastic seedling trays both with and without holes on the bottom. Standard size trays are 11 by 11 and 11 by 21 inches. Choose the size that best suits your location and your volume needs. Three trays are required to build one grower—two without holes, and one with holes.

Step 1. Soak Seeds. Soak your wheat berries in a large jar of pure water for 9–12 hours. Initially you will need to determine how much to soak by laying one level of dry seed into the bottom of the tray. Just cover the bottom once—don't double it. Keep that measure for future reference. Again, seed quality makes all the difference growing good wheatgrass. Review our previous seed suggestions.

Step 2. Germinate. Pour the berries (ideally) into a hemp sprouting bag (see Resources) and germinate them for two days. Transplant to the tray when the shoots are about twice the length of the berry and each seed exhibits several long, hairlike roots.

Step 3. Transplant. Pick up the tray with the holes on the bottom and pour the seeds into it. If too many of the sprouts fall through the holes, then you need to germinate one more day in the sprout bag. Some seed loss is acceptable.

Step 4. Grow and Rinse. Rinse the seedlings gently with a shower spray being careful not to shove the seeds out of their positions. You may already have a dish spray hose that is built into your sink. Use it or buy a faucet spray adaptor from the hardware store. Do not mist with a spray bottle. Misting does not provide the necessary water pressure to wash away waste and bacteria. This begins your routine of rinsing twice per day (or more in very hot weather). Remember—the sprouts prefer to be showered rather than drilled with the jet of a faucet.

Step 5. Set in Base. Take the solid bottom tray and place four corks near the corners. Nest the tray of seedlings inside the solid bottom tray and set it on the four corks. The corks provide an airspace separation of approximately three quarters (¾) of an inch. You can choose to use something else–like wood–however, cork does not mold.

Step 6. The Greenhouse. Now grab the second tray with the solid bottom and place it inverted on top of the seedlings tray. Locate the grower in a spot convenient to the sink. That's all until the evening, when the rinsing routine repeats.

The purpose of rinsing is to cool down the sprouts and wash off any waste or bacteria. Adequate rinsing eliminates mold and other common problems. Spend at least 30 seconds watering your sprouts with a strong shower of water, but not so strong that it rearranges the position of the seeds. Again, refer to the soil-growing instructions for all other gardening issues including light, water, temperature, etc.

Growing Other Sprouts with This Method

Green pea shoots, buckwheat, and sunflower greens will also grow successfully in this sprouter following the same instructions. Green pea shoots grow 10 inches tall in approximately 9 days. You can use either green or red peas. Buckwheat takes approximately 12 days. Use only the black, unhulled grain. They are mature when at least 80% of the black hulls have fallen off and their clover-like leaves have unfolded. Sunflower also takes about 12 days and is ready when 80% of the shells have dropped, revealing a hearty "V" shaped sprout. To harvest, grab a small bunch and gently wiggle them free or cut them just above the roots.

Cost Comparison: Buying vs. Growing			
	Purchase Price per bottle or tray	#Servings Serving Size	Cost per Serving
Purchase Grown Grass[1]	$15.00 lb	10	$1.50
Barley Grass Juice[2] Powder	$33 @5.3oz	50 @3g	$0.66
Wheat Grass Juice[3] Powder	$57 @8oz	76 @3g	$0.75
Whole Grass Powdered[4]	$56 @24oz	227 @3g	$0.25
Juice Bar Grass Juice	$1.75 @1oz	1 @ 1oz	$1.75
Home Grown & Juiced	$1.80/lb/tray	10	$0.18

1. Mail order shipped grass. 2. Green Magma. 3. Pines juice powder. 4. Pines whole leaf powder. Prices may increase over the years, but the relative costs should hold true.

How Much Does It Cost?

There is no question that growing your own grass is more economical than having someone else grow it for you. But the low cost of getting juice from your own crop may be somewhat deceiving. The hidden cost is in the labor and equipment. The price of your time, materials, and juicing machine are hard to calculate. But if you add them up, they make the juice bar and powdered grass alternatives more attractive. Unfortunately, fresh wheat wheatgrass from juice bars or health stores is not available everywhere. If you are unlucky with your location, then you could dial a toll-free number and have your grass delivered tomorrow. The *Resource* chapter lists several vendors that offer this service. That eliminates the growing— now all you have to do is the juicing! But mail order may not be cost effective if you are a volume user or on a budget. If you are a volume user, you may have little choice but to grow your own or hire a gardener.

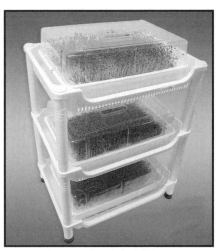

A commercial soil-free
wheatgrass grower

The alternatives? You can use the finest powdered grasses in combination with fresh vegetable juice (see *Healing* and *The Companies* chapters). Refer to the *Resources* chapter for the latest alternative wheatgrass products. The convenience and portability of the powdered juices is very attractive. But the cost of growing, juicing, dehydrating, and packaging is dear. These production costs are simply not present when growing your own grass. When all the calculations are done, it turns out that whether you grow soil-free or in soil, homegrown is still dirt cheap. At only pennies per ounce, you can guzzle enough of your own stash to keep you in-the-green for a long time.

The Juicers

This chapter introduces you to some of the equipment necessary to make your own fresh squeezed wheatgrass juice. Since your health depends on it, you will want to choose carefully and explore all the options. Most of the juicers described here will also juice fruit and vegetables. A versatile juicer will become, without question, the most important nutritional appliance in your kitchen. As a dispenser of vitamins and minerals alone, this machine will provide hundreds of dollars worth of savings. And that does not count all the fun you and your family will have using it. A juicer is a magic thirst-quenching, fountain-of-youth machine that conjures up all kinds of flavors and colors to interest even the most soda-pop minded family member. If you are committed to the pursuit of health, get a good juicing machine and watch it become your personal drug store and medicine chest for all that ails you.

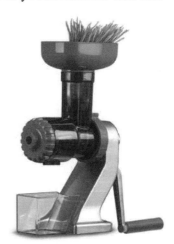

The Z-Star by Tribest. A modern plastic manual wheatgrass juicer

Wheatgrass juicers are very versatile. Because they operate by grinding, pressing, and extruding, they can extract the juice from any leafy green vegetable—one of the hardest jobs for any juicing machine. Most of these machines will juice any fruit or vegetable you can stick in them. In addition, they will grind nuts and seeds into butters such as peanut butter, almond butter, sunflower meal, and sesame butter to name a few. Some machines even offer attachments for making flour and extruding different shapes of pasta. But perhaps their most popular feature is making frozen fruit custards. It's easy. Just freeze your favorite berry and push them through the juicer alternating with frozen bananas. Out comes an extruded, custard-like frozen dessert that is a winner with kids of all ages and at any party.

This chapter is not a Consumer Reports review. Brands are not discussed and compared. Instead the goal of this chapter is to explain and introduce the different categories of juicers so that you can make an informed decision and purchase the juicing machine that best suits your philosophy and budget. No brand preferences are stated or implied, but you can get a complete list of juicer manufacturers in the *Resources* chapter. Request their brochures and try to buy from vendors you trust.

Why Common Juicers and Blenders Won't Work

All juicers are not equal. You can buy a juicer from Wal-Mart for under $100, but it definitely won't juice wheatgrass. These machines are usually products of large, general appliance manufacturers some of whom are more famous for video games and portable stereos. Most of these machines are centrifuges that spin at high velocities of 3,000 revolutions per minute (rpms). They have weak motors and if you put anything in them more complicated than a stalk of celery, they fume and squawk and dance around the counter damaging themselves and anything in their path.

What to Shop for in A Juicer

- Ability to Extract Nutrients
- Convenience of operation
- Ease of Assembly
- Size and space
- Price

- Durability
- Powerful Motor
- Pulp Disposal Method
- Efficiency of Clean-up
- Length of Warranty

A wheatgrass juicer is actually a screw press. It presses and squeezes the pulp, much like the old fashioned washboards that twist and wring out the wetness from your laundry. This process is sometimes called trituration or mastication. These are fancy words that basically describe the squeezing and grinding action of a worm gear or auger. They tear and rip the vegetable fibers apart releasing the phytonutrients from the plant cells. In contrast, centrifugal juicers don't get past the cell walls. They slice the vegetable fibers into tiny fractions. You get the nutrition between the cells but not from within. These machines are in no way designed to handle the woody, ligneous fibers of grass. It would be like sticking a branch with leaves into your blender. If that weren't bad enough, their high speeds oxidize and destroy the enzymes and bio-active ingredients that make wheatgrass so therapeutic. When it comes to juicing wheatgrass or any other leafy vegetable—parsley, spinach, lettuce, celery, herbs and sprouts—high speed, centrifugal force juicers are verboten.

And while we are talking speed, don't even think about buying a blender. Blenders don't juice anything—no fruits, no vegetables. But when it comes to wheatgrass, it gets even worse. The grass blades will wrap around the steel blades and strangle your blender to death. Even if your blender survives, the high speed action aerates, oxidizes, and heats up the grass. That's bad enough but worse you get about one-tenth the volume you would otherwise produce in a wheatgrass juicer. Even the famous Vita-Mix, the all powerful multi-purpose kitchen appliance, is neither designed for nor recommended for juicing wheatgrass. Don't compromise. The goal is not to minimize the number of appliances in your kitchen. It is to maximize the nutrients extracted from your produce.

The Original Wheatgrass Juicer

When Ann Wigmore started looking for a way to juice her grass, she grabbed a cast iron tin-plated meat grinder. It almost worked, but it did not separate the pulp. Back in the middle 1960s, there were still a few cast iron foundries remaining in the U.S. They made meat grinders and berry presses. These worm gear, screw-press hand grinders had been crushing and squeezing berries and nuts for generations. The addition of a stainless steel screen enabled these presses to capture the juice and separate it from the grass pulp. The pressure can be adjusted via a screw on the front to make your grass drier. All units were cast iron with heavy duty, hot dip tin plating (except in grinding areas). They clamped onto the counter and they worked. But it took a couple of minutes of hand cranking to make one ounce and you need 10 to 20 ounces daily if you are trying to cure something.

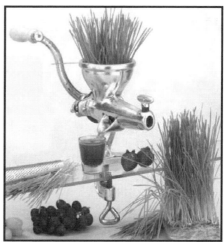

Along came Adlen Link from New York who figured out a way to motorize the manual juicer and thereby invented the first electric wheatgrass juicer. He made so many for Dr. Ann and her Hippocrates Institute clients that he started his own company called Sundance. This was the original wheatgrass juicer

A popular cast iron manual wheatgrass juicer manufactured by Miracle Exclusives.

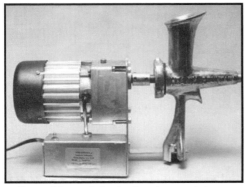
One of the original wheatgrass juicers
developed by Sundance

and Alden's design remained the prototype for all wheatgrass juicers for the next thirty years.

The early machines worked well, but they were definitely not mainstream. They were wobbly, noisy, and messy. Their main disadvantage came at clean-up time. Cast iron rusts and needs to be oiled or "cured" just like the old cast iron skillets. This is just one more chore for the already busy wheatgrass user. It was okay in the early days, but as the wheatgrass world expanded, users chose rust-free juicing and easy clean-up.

The Twin Gear Juicers

When the *Green Power Juice Extractor* came along in 1994, it instantly became the most exciting entry on the juicer playing field in decades. With its patented invention of two juicing augers, it was both innovative and unique. It was also avant-garde. Lodged inside its twin stainless steel gears, there are magnets and ceramics that produce positive ions as the gears spin. According to the designers, this effect reduces the wear and tear of oxidation thereby increasing the longevity of the juice. The juice lasts longer because more enzymes and nutrients remain intact enhancing stability. Users claim that carrot juice can be refrigerated for 48 hours. Although drinking the fresh juice immediately is best, increasing the staying power of the juice means you can juice once per day instead of twice. Anything that can save the chore of juicing increases the potential for more drinks and thus the therapeutic benefit.

One of the main advantages of this juicer is its versatility. It will juice carrots and wheatgrass at the same time. Traditionally, these two required different machines. Juicing carrots right along with your wheatgrass is wonderful for both taste and convenience and may persuade even the most reluctant wheatgrass drinkers. It also juices sprouts, herbs, grasses, leafy greens, apples— basically all popular vegetables and fruits. Use this same machine to entertain non-wheatgrass guests with nut butters, frozen fruit sorbets, mochi (Japanese rice cakes) and 3 different shapes of pasta.

The twin stainless steel gears spin at a slow 90 rpms, crushing the vegetables and forcing out the juice against a fine sieve. The slow rotation means no oxidation and no friction as compared to the 3,000 rpms of the centrifugal juicers. Since it is also a pulp ejector (ejects the pulp immediately rather than collects it), you can juice continuously without stopping to clean. When you do need to clean up, there are five parts to wash and remount: the two gears, the strainer, and front and back housing. Because there are two gears, there is one more part to assemble and clean than with the more common single auger juicers. But the twin gears are considered the smoothest and quietest machines available. When the twin gears came on the market, they eliminated the maddening noise, heat, and vibration that had been a part of the juicing process for decades. Whoever designed the original twin gear juicer, was a very creative individual and also a dedicated juice lover. This is evident in the use of magnets, the slow turning gears, the one-machine-juices-all design, the multi-purpose appliance functions, the low noise, and even the sturdy built-in handle for moving and storing. No surprise that when it premiered, it won the Silver medal prize at the International Exhibition of Inventions in Germany. Today, there are a few twin gear machines on the market. Prices range from $400 to $600 US.

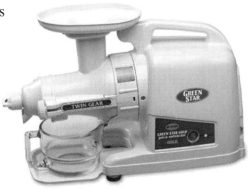

The original twin gear wheatgrass juicer first imported into the U.S. by Tribest in 1994

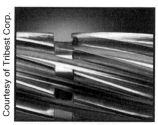

Courtesy of Tribest Corp.

Stainless steel gears provide long life and the highest quality extraction

The Single Gear Juicers

Twin gear juicers are without question the gold standard for juicing wheatgrass and all fruits and vegetables. But when the single gear machines were introduced, they offered something else—high end performance in a compact size at a low price. That's hard to beat. Sure, you get one gear instead of two, plastic instead of stainless steel, less motor and less torque, but that is where the sacrifice ends. You still get the capacity to juice wheatgrass and all fruits and vegetables. You still get the slow turning, no-oxidation technology. And you still get the versatility to make custards and pastas.

The best news about these juicers is the price. Thanks to good old fashioned competition, these machines sell in the $200 to $300 US price range. And there are many to choose from. Of course, there are differences between the brands, but the features are generally the same. Some models are so similar, their parts can be exchanged and still fit in the competitors machine. If you are going to choose a single gear juicer, take a good look at the auger itself and the screen. These are the essential elements. Beyond that, consider the company you are purchasing from, the warranty, and the after purchase customer service.

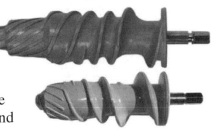

Photo by Tribest Corp.

Not all single gear augers are created equal.

These are pulp ejector juicers, so you can juice all day without stopping to clean. Assembly and cleaning of the various modes are essentially equal. They have the same number of parts: the gear, the strainer, the housing, and the end nozzle. A sieve is often included to reduce any excess pulp that makes it through the strainer. A nozzle at the end can also be changed to match the food being juiced. Tightening the knob squeezes out more juice, loosening it increases the rate of flow. As with the twin gear juicers, there is a great escape feature in case you overstuff your machine—a reverse button. Because wheatgrass juicers are slow turning machines (80 revolutions per minute) they can get bogged down with compacted pulp, occasionally forcing you to disassemble the machine. But the reverse motor feature will get you out of a jam. Single gear machines are your best choice if you are on a budget.

Choose a machine that matches your lifestyle and budget and is manageable for you to use on a regular basis.

The Final Analysis

There is no free-ride in the world of juicing. All juicers must be assembled and disassembled for each use. Although this is a consideration, all the machines described here basically demand the same amount of work.

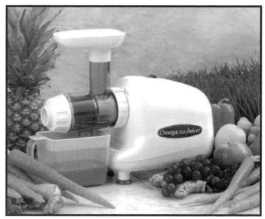

They all have an auger gear or two, a cover, a screen, a nozzle, and a juicer housing, all of which must be cleaned and assembled. You can compare the differences in handling these parts from one machine to another ad infinitum, but in the end, the speed and efficiency of your clean-up and assembly chores depend more on your establishing a routine and developing shortcuts than anything else.

A popular single gear juicer manufactured by Omega. Single gear juicers provide high end performance at an economical price.

Finally, whatever juicer you choose, it all squeezes down to this: Will you use it? The cold facts about owning a wheatgrass juicer or any kind of juicer are size, space, and convenience of operation. Why are these so important? Because if you become discouraged by any of these factors, you will use it less. An unused juicer does nothing for your health. Choose a machine that matches your lifestyle and budget and is manageable for you to use on a regular basis. Regular use is the secret to unleashing the power of juice therapy.

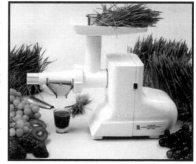

One of the best selling wheatgrass juicers ever, by Miracle Exclusives

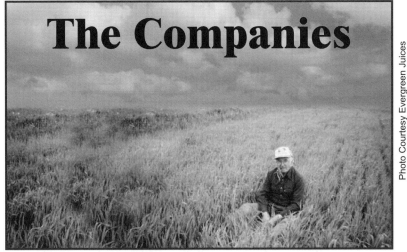

Greet the Products You'll Meet
on the Store Shelves

Choose the best grass products to fit your diet and lifestyle

This chapter will introduce you to the grass companies you'll meet on your health food store shelves. It is not a complete list of all manufacturers. However, it does include the major producers who grow and process the grasses that end up in the products you see. Keep in mind that many brands are just repackagers of the products grown by the companies listed here. These companies are chosen because they actually grow the product, harvest, and bottle it. Although it cannot possibly include everyone, it does provide a mix that represents the marketplace. Here, you will find the full range of manufacturers: Those who grow outdoors and in, who make frozen and fresh, juice and whole leaf, the private labelers and the self-branded. New growers are "sprouting" up all the time. So, for the latest information, see the *Resources* chapter and visit the website for this book at www.Sproutman.com. The following pages will give you a good idea of what goes into the grass you drink and what goes on behind-the-scenes. It is intended to help you make informed purchasing decisions relating to quality, ethics, organic-ness, processing methods, etc. This background information also gives you a sense of a company's philosophy so you can match your inclinations to theirs. No recommendations are intended,1 and the listing sequence is entirely arbitrary. Neither the author nor publisher receive financial benefit from any of these companies.

However, the author has used all of the products, and visited, met, or spoken with the principals of all the companies. In short, you cannot go wrong with any of these products. And if you fancy yourself a connoisseur, you might try them all! You are sure to get healthier with every drink. The goal of this chapter is to help you find the best product (for you), and the easiest way to include grass in your diet.

Field Growers or Tray Growers?

Do you think that wheatgrass is supposed to be grown in trays? Well, not exactly...Ann Wigmore popularized the growing of wheatgrass indoors because she lived in a major city in the wintry northeast. What was her alternative? Years later, when asked why she didn't grow outdoors, she reportedly answered: "Well, I never thought of it." Wheatgrass actually started as an outdoor grown product. (Makes sense doesn't it.) That was the grass that rejuvenated the sick chickens in the 1930s. (See *The Pioneers, Schnabel.*)

Field growers have hundreds of acres to manage. They cut their grass at a low eight to ten inches and before the jointing stage that Charles Schnabel defined. If temperatures are warm, growth can progress quickly, and farmers are hard pressed to harvest their crop in such a short time. However, they must meet the task or lose their investment. Growers must be diligent about capturing the plant at this peak time of maximum nutrition and then protect it right through the harvesting, drying, milling and packaging. If this weren't hard enough, field growers are forever challenged by weather. If it is too hot, too cold, too rainy or too dry, there is trouble. It is not unusual for a farmer to lose fifty acres of beautiful wheat, just because the ground was too wet to send out the harvesters. By the time things dry up, the grain may have matured beyond the jointing stage and it's just too late. As much as two hundred days of growing can be lost! As you will learn in this chapter, most of the major wheatgrass companies are field growers. Worldwide there are a couple dozen of them. But tray growers are a different story. There are hundreds of them. Search the *Resources* chapter for the one closest to you. A round of applause please, for all the hard working farmers, both indoors and out.

Green*Life*™

V.E. Irons. Sonne's Organic Foods, Inc. Kansas City, Missouri
800-544-8147, fax 1-816-221-1272 www.sonnes.com

No one seems to realize that to produce Greenlife we use more fuel for heating, condensing, and refrigeration than most large hospitals. All this is necessary for one purpose only —to retain the life in the product. —V.E. Irons

This is the company that health pioneer V.E. Irons founded in 1946 and it is the oldest existing grass foods producer in the world. (See *The Pioneers*.) Their product, **Green*life*™** has been marketed since 1951. It is the dried extracted juice of organically grown cereal grasses: barley, oats, rye, and wheat. The grasses are grown on 575 acres along the Gasconade River on rich Missouri soil. In fact, the town's name is *Richland*, Missouri. They use biodynamic methods, which is a specialized organic practice. But they have not signed on to the organic certification program. "We've been organic since before they even thought of it!" says Julia Irons. The processing plant is located at the farm. The grass is ground, the juice is extracted using a giant, slow turning twin gear style juicer that looks like a nine-foot long Greenstar. (See *The Juicers*) The chilled juice is then dried in a roll-dryer inside a vacuum chamber at a low 90°F. The dried grass comes out like crepe paper and is then pressed into tablets. This company prefers tablets because the powder readily absorbs moisture, which turns it brown and gummy. Moisture is so critical at this stage that their powder room was designed with six inches of insulation on the walls to keep out the humidity. The product is then inserted into dark brown glass bottles with loosely covered caps and placed into a nitrogen chamber where the oxygen is drawn out of the bottle and replaced with nitrogen.

Products

This is an old fashioned "health" company. Their products are neither fancy, nor commercial in design, nor conventionally marketed. They promote health first and the products are simply tools for health. V.E. Irons is famous for his philosophy of colon cleansing to achieve optimum health. All of this company's products fit under the theme of detoxification and intestinal cleansing. Its flagship product is a seven day cleansing kit with psyllium seed bulk fiber and liquid bentonite detoxificant. Greenlife (also part of this kit) fits perfectly into the colon health regimen because it bathes the intestines with chlorophyll and nutrition. Greenlife is ninety-two percent grass from wheat, barley, oats, and rye. The remainder is from beets and sea kelp. This is a "juice powder" with the grass fiber removed. They also manufacture a "fortified" version which combines Greenlife, sixty percent, with fish liver oils, brewers yeast, papain, bone meal, and lecithin (not a vegetarian product). They sell direct to consumers under the "Vitratox" brand, which stands for vitamins, minerals, and detoxification (the original line sold by V.E. Irons in 1952) and in health food stores under the name Sonne Organic Foods.

> *It would be so much easier to dry the grass in its entirety, pulverize it and sell you hay in ground form, or perhaps tray dry and spray dry the grass juice. The analysis might be the same but there is no life!. Remember, Live foods produce Live Tissue—Dead foods produce Dead tissue.* —V.E. Irons

Pines Wheatgrass

Pines International. 1-800-MY-PINES, fax 785-841-1252
Lawrence, Kansas   www.Wheatgrass.com

> *Cereal grass is easy to grow. Whether or not it provides high nutritional concentration depends on where you grow it, when you harvest it and how you store and process it.* —Ron Seibold

Pines is the largest wheat grass grower in the world. Started in 1976, Pines carries on the tradition of Dr. Charles Schnabel, the original pioneer of wheatgrass (see *The Pioneers*), who first used it as a source of human food. Its founders, Ron Seibold and Steve Malone were not originally farmers or businessmen. The concepts that launched this company were mostly social and environmental and they still live up to those principles. Both were disappointed with the increase in chemical agriculture and the rape of the land by corporate developers. Growing cereal grass and selling it provided a way to earn money and preserve land at the same time. They saw Pines as an opportunity to stay connected to the land they grew up on and work with some of their neighbors to develop a sustainable community. The name "Pines" was chosen because it is considered the international symbol of peace in nature. Seibold and Malone started the company with small ($100) stock purchases from their own pockets, and those of their employees and farmers. It is still cooperatively owned today by its

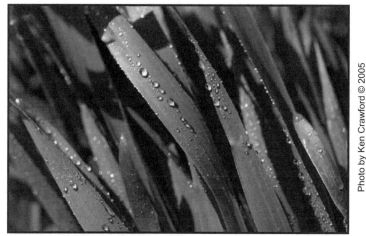

Pines Wheatgrass, Lawrence, Kansas

original founders, stockholders, farmers, neighbors, and employees—truly a grass roots company!

Today, Pines owns 2,000 acres of rich, certified organic Kansas land—all of which has been converted from pesticides and herbicides. The company has committed much of its after-tax-profits to land preservation projects. In addition, they have an International Hunger Relief program in which they donate the grass foods they harvest to the needy worldwide. Since 1991, over three million dollars worth of cereal grass foods have been contributed to Native Americans and the homeless in the U.S., and to organizations that distribute food for famine relief in Africa, Central America, Asia, Korea and Europe. Pines has also established a Wilderness Community Education Foundation on their land and constructed three energy-efficient demonstration homes.

How The Grass is Grown

Kansas provides an ideal climate for growing grasses. Pines plants in the fall and harvests in the spring. During the approximately 200 days in between, the grass develops deep mature roots which pull minerals from the rich soil and send it up to the leaves in the spring. Pines makes sure to provide those minerals by rotating the wheat fields with soybeans and red clover. Harvest time in April is short and feverish. According to the research done by Charles Schnabel, the father of wheatgrass, the grass must be harvested just before the jointing stage when the plant commits

its stored nutrition to the development of the seed head (grain). After jointing, wheat grows rapidly and its nutrient concentration drops precipitously *(see Jointing, p. 43)*. When harvested, the grass is only about seven to ten inches tall but the root systems, buried well below the frost line, are twelve inches or more.

Harvesting and Processing

Growing healthy grass on good organic land is not enough. The grass must be harvested, dried, ground, tableted, stored and packaged. Meticulous attention has to be given to each phase or the product will lose its bio-activity. Pines harvests using special custom-built harvesters with sterile collection hoppers. The machines cut only the top three inches or so from the seven to ten inch tall grass which is only harvested once. If they took a second cutting, grew it longer or cut it lower, they would reap greater volume and save production costs but at the sacrifice of nutrition. The remaining grass is thus left to continue to grow past the jointing stage to full maturity. Meanwhile, the harvester never lets the grass touch the ground, nor is it touched by human hands. The grass is very quickly transported from the harvester to the nearby dehydrator building. It is literally dried within minutes of harvest. Were it left lying on the ground waiting for delivery, it would bleach in the sun, oxidize and become contaminated. Their custom triple-bypass drum dehydrator dries the leaves in a mere two to three seconds with a core temperature that never exceeds 107°F. All this is done to maintain maximum nutritional integrity.

> *People are becoming more aware of the importance of darkgreen, leafy vegetables, but the traditional American diet doesn't include enough of them. Our products offer a convenient way to correct that deficiency without having to change your whole diet.* —Ron Seibold

From the dehydrator, the grass is pelletized to cut down on the surface area exposed to the elements. The pellets are stored in huge, nitrogen-filled pharmaceutical bags. Each bag holds a ton of grass pellets. The bags are stored in underground caves at 10°F until ready for tableting. Samples of every batch are tested for contamination by microbes and for nutritional value. When needed, the grass is removed from storage for processing into powder or tablets. The milling or fine grinding of the grass is done so there is no heat to destroy product vitality. Tablets and powder are then packed in amber glass bottles in a vacuum chamber where all oxygen is removed and replaced by nitrogen. This enables long shelf life and prevents deterioration and oxidation from exposure to air and light.

I pulled a test on myself to make sure the wheatgrass was actually helping me. I quit taking it. In two months time, I can tell you that physically it made a difference. People have even noticed a difference in my skin and eyes.[2]

Products and Fiber

Pines manufactures a full line of cereal grasses including wheat, barley, oat, and alfalfa. Their flagship products are 100 percent whole leaf dried grasses of wheat and barley in powder or tablets. No fillers, binders, or other ingredients are used. To a lesser extent, they also offer "juice powders" in which the grass is juiced and then spray dried. But Pines prefers to promote the consumption of grasses as whole fiber vegetables instead of juice. They proclaim the many proven benefits of vegetable fiber and the shortage of it in the American diet. Furthermore, fiber carries some nutrients which are lost when it's removed. Not only does their grass provide the benefits of fiber, but it is very economical, offering a full serving of green vegetables for as little as twenty cents per serving. Their combination product is called *Mighty Greens* and is a blend of wheat, barley, oat and rye grasses, alfalfa, spirulina, chlorella, royal jelly, and sixteen other herbs and superfoods. Their website is the famous Wheatgrass.com. You can read Ron Seibold's thoroughly researched book, *Cereal Grasses*, online there and they welcome your email questions and comments.

We don't take out what nature puts in. —Ron Seibold

Green Magma®

Green Foods Corporation. Oxnard, California

800-777-4430, fax 805-983-8843 www.greenfoods.com

Green Foods Corporation is the largest of the grass producers with divisions in both the US and Japan. Yoshihide Hagiwara, its founder, is a living legend and pioneer of barley grass (See *The Pioneers*). Although wheatgrass has the name recognition, many claim that barley is the superior of these two triticum brothers. This company is a major marketing

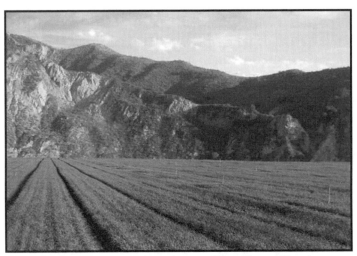

Barley grass growing at one of the Green Foods
Corporation farms in Ventura county California

force behind the green foods revolution. It is the only grass manufacturer that has run advertising on national cable networks such as the *Discovery Channel, The Learning Channel* and *Lifetime*. At various times, they have used endorsements from professional athletes including golf legend Arnold Palmer, and doctors. Dr. James Balch, co-author of the best seller *Prescription for Nutritional Healing* said: "The variety of vitamins and minerals found in barley essence is unmatched by any other single fruit or vegetable."

More than any other company, Green Foods Corp (GFC) has put its money into research. Hagiwara, a pharmacist and researcher himself, is president of the Hagiwara Institute for Nutritional Research in Tokyo and has financed research at major Universities in the USA and Japan. While the therapeutic benefits of wheatgrass has depended primarily on clinical evidence and testimonials, Hagiwara and GFC have made substantial inroads into legitimizing the value of grass foods in the eyes of science and medicine.

Dr. Takayuki Shibamoto, Ph.D., is a professor and former chair for the department of Environmental Toxicology at the University of California-Davis. He has isolated a powerful antioxidant isoflavonoid in young barley leaves called 2"-*0*-GIV. He claims that it helps lower cholesterol and is a better antioxidant than Vitamin C. He has published over 200 scientific papers and is the author of *A Strong Antioxidant Found in Young Green Barley Leaves*. Dr. Kazuhiko Kubota, Ph.D., is the author of

Studies on the Effects of Green Barley Juice on the Endurance and Motor Activity in Mice. He has performed extensive research on barley leaf extract and discovered many pharmacological functions including anti-inflammation, anti-ulcer, lowering of blood sugar levels, and increased endurance. He is chairman of the Department of Pharmacy at the Science University of Tokyo. (See *Nutrition & Research*)

In spite of all this research, GFC makes no claims about their product in relation to specific diseases. Their stated purpose is prevention and the intent of their marketing efforts is to provide a product that is convenient to use and appeals to the mass market.

Growing, Harvesting & Processing

GFC is located near the Pacific coast on the beautiful Oxnard plains famous for being the world capital of strawberries. Its organic growing fields are located further north in the more pristine, remote environment in Eastern Ventura Country, California. For eons, rain draining off the adjacent mountains has delivered its mineral rich content to the plains. Over time, lots of silt has built up there and it has become home to turf farms raising marathon turf. Because the Pacific coast climate is so favorable, the grass can be grown year-round. Every sixty days organically raised barley leaves are harvested at the jointing stage. Two cuttings are taken from each field. Within forty-five minutes the grass

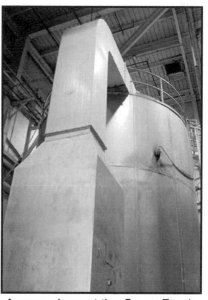

A spray dryer at the Green Foods Corporation plant.

is delivered to the 52,000 square foot processing facility. This is a massive, super-efficient, state-of-the-art plant that is truly impressive.

The grass is first washed thoroughly, rinsed and tumble dried without the use of chemicals, heat or detergents. Then the leaves are sent through a corkscrew press to gently extract the juice. The insoluble plant fiber is returned to the fields where it is mixed with natural fertilizers for compost. The juice is concentrated and ready for spray drying after it is combined with maltodextrin and brown rice. Both these serve as a carriers and binders for the powder. The huge computer controlled spray drier is a patented invention of Hagiwara designed to keep heat sensitive enzymes alive. It sprays the juice into a fine mist of dried powder at a temperature that never exceeds 98°F. The powder is then protected from oxidation, granulated and packaged. The plant has four quality control engineers on duty. Every lot is inspected for microbes and evaluated for nutrient content including enzymatic activity.

Just the Juice. Not the Fiber

There are two camps among the manufacturers in the grass industry—those that juice the grass and dry it into a powder and those that take the whole leaf and powder that. GFC is a juice company. While they acknowledge the value of dietary fiber, that is not the purpose of this product. Anyone who wants more fiber in their diet has numerous foods to choose from. Hagiwara created a precious vitamin concentrate that he designed to be fully assimilated, not slowed down or blocked by the various inefficiencies of people's digestive tracts. He tells us that fiber is indigestible and locks some nutrients inside it whereas juice is fully soluble and instantly assimilable even by people with weak digestion.

The Story Behind Maltodextrin

This is the most controversial subject about GFC and all of its detractors readily jump on it. Unfortunately, consumers know little about the pros and cons of the various additives in foods and don't take the time to investigate. Once they hear something negative, it usually sticks. Here's the story on maltodextrin. It is a complex carbohydrate derived from potato starch or corn. Carbohydrates are sugars and starches from foods like grains, and vegetables like potatoes and squash. Complex carbohydrates take longer to enter the bloodstream, while simpler sugars enter rapidly, causing the roller coaster energy highs and lows that hypoglycemics well know. Because maltodextrin is complex, it is safe for diabetics. It does not spike blood sugar. It is used in the spray drying process because Hagiwara discovered that it encapsulates enzymes and nutrients protecting them from oxidation. It is especially helpful in preventing the degradation of chlorophyll that breaks down into toxic pheophorbide if oxidized. Maltodextrin makes up about thirty percent of the formula and brown rice another five percent. (The company won't confirm.) Some people are dismayed by this, but here are a few points to consider. Tray grown grass has proven its therapeutic benefits to thousands of people. Yet it naturally contains about sixty percent simple sugars. Magma contains thirty percent complex sugars and it also works. Indeed, it is the most researched grass product on the market. Sometimes there are tradeoffs in a less than perfect world, and we as consumers need to make decisions. If this additive preserves nutrients and enhances flavor and enzymatic activity, is that a good value? It's your choice.

Green Foods Corporation has a whole family of Magma products including *Magma Plus*, a superfoods combo product, barley grass formulas for your pets, and *Veggie-Magma* that includes juices from vegetables and sprouts.

Dynamic Greens Wheatgrass

16128 Ninth Line, Stouffville, Ontario Canada

877-910-0467, 905-910-0467. www.dynamicgreens.com

The Beginning

How does a wheatgrass farm start? When Janice Stem was diagnosed with breast cancer in 1972, the family adopted the Ann Wigmore program of growing wheatgrass in trays in the kitchen. But as the years went by, Janice developed allergies. Her allergic reaction was a throaty croupy cough that would last for an hour or two after drinking wheatgrass juice. When they experimented with outdoor grown wheatgrass, Janice had no reaction. Upon examining the indoor grass they found a tiny white fuzz near the soil—mold. They tried cutting above the white fuzz, and although it helped, Janice still had a little reaction. They had forty trays growing indoors for years, but this forced them to look at outdoor grass as an alternative. They started growing in a small twenty-by-fifty foot section. But by 1983, other people were also using their wheatgrass, and that space just kept expanding. Their growing season was mid-May to early November. With winter approaching, they had to make a decision. How could they provide a continuous wheatgrass juice source with outdoor grown grass? Since the outdoor grass did not seem to mind the frost, their solution was to preserve the grass by freezing. (For more on Janice Stem's story, *see p. 107.*) They drank frozen juice for six months and switched to fresh outdoor wheatgrass in the Spring.

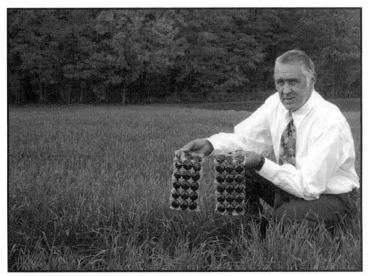

Farmer and founder Tom Stem in his field of young
wheatgrass holding his sealed packages of grass juice.

Farmer and founder Tom Stem cuts the grass at a height of six to ten inches, which represents about two months growth in the outdoor environment. They harvest from May through November. Although they harvest right through the hot summer, grass likes the cold. The grass they plant in October is not harvested until May. This is called "winter wheat" because the grass sleeps over the winter. During this time, the grass is basically under the snow. Its roots grow long, nourishing the grass and keeping it warm. When the grass is harvested in May, it is only four to six inches tall!

> *Quality, not quantity is the principle behind these decisions*
> *because people are depending on this for their medicine.*
> —Tom Stem, founder, Dynamic Greens

Attention to Detail At Every Step

As you can see, a great deal of attention is paid to the growing. But even good grass can be ruined on its way to the juicer. So care and attention must be paid to every step. Harvesting is one of those crucial steps. Using a rotary mower, for example, bruises the grass terribly. The Stems use a sickle type blade that runs back and forth between teeth. It just snips it. There is no bruising and no signs of oxidation. The cut grass is carried to the trailer behind the mower by a conveyer belt, not blown through a chute. The trailer then heads to the juicing room, which is right on the property. During harvest time, there are ten to twenty people working; they mow, load the trailer, wash, juice, package, and freeze. All these steps must be orchestrated simultaneously. Timing is crucial to maximizing quality.

Juicing

First the grass is chilled by washing it in cold water. It is not a bath because that leeches nutrients by osmosis. Instead the grass travels slowly under a row of nozzles showering them with a strong spray. The conveyer belt also vibrates to shake off excess water. It arrives at the juicing machine washed and dried. Dynamic Greens made their own juicing machine that uses two gears to squash the grass, and press out its juice. It operates like a giant twin gear home juicer *(see p. 179)*. Stainless steel gears compress the grass, then force the juice out through a strainer. The gears turn slowly so as not to create friction or oxidation.

Packaging and Freezing

Dynamic Greens package is a kind of skinny, flexible ice cube tray. But instead of square cubes, there are eighteen round bubbles each filled with .56 ounces—a little more than half an ounce of juice. They overfill a little so the total package yields approximately ten ounces of juice. Keeping bubbles out of the package is tricky business but it is essential because air deteriorates the juice. Air is the enemy of enzymes. Tom Stem says: "after all the hard work of growing, harvesting, cleaning, and juicing, we don't want to lose it now to oxidation."

> *As we go on, we make little improvements that shorten the time between harvest and juicing or speed up the freezing. Even if we just gain a few seconds, that could make all the difference in someone's struggle to restore their health.* —Tom Stem

The juice packages are then taken into the custom built walk-in freezer and placed on a rack. Cold air circulates above and below the rows of sealed grass packages. Double compressors provide a very quick freeze and also a backup in case one unit fails. The first batch in the morning freezes solid as a rock within ten minutes. As the day goes on and the freezer fills up, it naturally takes longer to go from liquid to ice. At that time, they bring in dry ice to accelerate the freezing. They get close to the freezing point in ten minutes, but it takes longer to harden.

Dynamic Greens is not sold in stores. Their product is shipped directly to individual homes. They send it out packed in a custom made styrofoam box with two inch thick walls. They offer either 120 or 240 ounces at a time and they ship overnight throughout the US and Canada for a flat fee.

Green Kamut®

Pure Planet. Long Beach, California. 800-695-2017
562-951-1124, Fax 562-951-5040. www.pureplanet.com

People examine purity first and price second. If the technology exists to dry grass without additives, then a 100% pure juice extract is clearly the superior choice. —David Sandoval

This company, under the guidance of entrepreneur David Sandoval, has virtually single-handedly pioneered the use of Kamut® wheat as an alternative to regular wheatgrass. Kamut® (*kamut.com*) is a variety of wheat that is superior to common wheat in protein and fatty acids. It is an ancient relative of modern durum wheat that originated in the fertile crescent of the Nile river thousands of years ago. The trademarked name[3] is the ancient Egyptian word for wheat whose root meaning is said to be "soul of the earth." It has only been grown in the U.S. since the 1980s. It is a non-hybrid, non crossbred seed internationally recognized as an heirloom grain. It is most famous for its rich buttery flavor, but you can even see the difference in its amber color and humped back kernel that is about twice the size of regular wheat. Although one might assume that genetically manipulated grain would be more nutritious, it is not the case. Instead the sad truth is that the thrust of modern agricultural engineering has been toward higher crop yields and the improvement of flour characteristics. Non-hybrid Kamut is actually more nutritious with about seventeen percent protein compared to an average twelve percent in common wheat. Sixteen out of eighteen of its amino acids rate higher than common wheat and it contains fourteen chromosome pairs compared to twenty-two in regular wheat. Kamut is also higher in eight out of nine minerals, contains more lipids and fatty acids and has significantly more magnesium, zinc and vitamin E.

How and Where It is Grown

The high mountains and ancient volcanic hills of Utah provide the ideal setting for the land where *Green Kamut* is grown. Their organic farm lies in a 5,000 foot high valley surrounded by canyons and mountains. Runoff from the mountains produced a lake thousands of years ago that still exists as a subterranean reservoir and provides a source of rich minerals for irrigation. Sandoval compares this mineral rich ancient seabed to the famous fertile crescent of the Nile, and says the top soil extends a deep eighteen feet. They grow "virgin grass" there, taking only one cutting at the jointing stage from each crop after approximately six weeks of growth. Each field grows alfalfa and Kamut on alternate years. This loads the soil with minerals and nitrogen that increases the chlorophyll content and the high altitude increases the protein. Green Kamut is actually a two ingredient product made up of sixty-five percent Kamut grass and thirty-five percent mature alfalfa. Alfalfa is loaded with minerals and is one of the richest sources of chlorophyll on the planet. This superb nutritional combination produces chlorophyll counts as high as two to three percent, which is equal to some algae. They also produce a 100 percent barley grass powder called *Just Barley*. Both of these products are highly alkaline forming foods, which is just what the bloodstream craves.

Processing and Packaging

Once the grass is harvested, it is washed and ground into a pulp. The pulp is chilled and juiced with a press. The moisture is then evaporated in a unique method that never exceeds 88°F., making this a non-pasteurized product. Their technique spreads out the molecules of the grass so it can dry quickly at a low temperature. This is the reason the product is so light-weight. The drier is heated by the company's new solar generator. The powder is then packaged in a plastic bottle with a desiccant pack to absorb moisture and sealed with a tamper proof lid. *Just Barley* is bottled in clear glass and protected from light by a display box made from recycled paper. No excipients, binders, fillers, starches or anti-caking agents are added to either product.

> *Scientists have discovered that green juices increase the oxygenation of the body, purify the blood and organs, aid in the metabolism of nutrients and counteract acids and toxins. Green juices are the superstars of the nutrition world.*
> —David Sandoval, Green Kamut

Sheldon Farm Wheatgrass

P.O Box 531 Chaplin, Connecticut

860-974-3375. 866-974-3375.   www.SheldonFarm.com

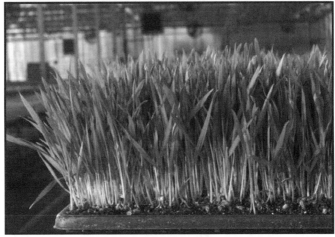

Grass grows mold-free in the Sheldon Farm greenhouse.

Sheldon Farms is the newest and smallest manufacturer of powdered grass and is unique in several ways. Compared with the outdoor producers, this grass is different in how it is grown and how it is dried. It looks and tastes different, too. They are currently the only bottled grass product manufacturer in distribution that does its growing in greenhouses— three of them to be exact. If you are a home grower, a connoisseur of juice bar wheatgrass, or a graduate of any of the wheatgrass retreat centers, this juice will taste like the fresh squeezed wheatgrass you are used to. It tastes completely different from any of the outdoor grown grass powder discussed in this chapter. This juice concentrate has that same sweet home-grown, fresh squeezed grass taste.

Growing & Juicing

Growing indoors has many differences over outdoor farming. Although this is not the place to discuss the pros and cons, (see *Nutrition* chapter) one of the biggest differences is in the management of the soil. Grower Mark Sheldon actually makes his own soil from five different ingredients including organic compost and rock dust powder—a highly concentrated source of minerals and trace minerals. In addition, he fertilizes with a proprietary eighty-eight mineral formula that includes microbes and enzymes. High protein organic wheat is sprouted in two inches of the special soil and watered with water from an artesian well. The grass is harvested at a height of six to eight inches and from eleven to fourteen days, depending on the season. And here's another advantage. There is no off-season. They can harvest all year round.

What farmer wouldn't want to control the weather! At Sheldon Farms, that is exactly what they do. Temperature and humidity in the greenhouse are automatically regulated according to the grower's settings. The quarter-acre sized greenhouse has sides that open and close as does the roof. This is how they control air circulation, temperature, and light. The roof is made out of a crystal clear poly-acrylic material called *Dynaglass* that blocks UV-A and UV-B rays. It has a slightly higher light transmission rating than glass, so you may feel the need for sunglasses inside but you could never get skin cancer. There are no grow lamps; only natural light. When it's winter, there is an energy-saving blanket that stretches across the growing area like a ten foot ceiling trapping the radiant heat and warming the grass significantly. The soil spreading and seed sowing are all done automatically enabling this operation to easily produce 1,000 trays per week or more if needed.

As soon as the grass is cut, it is juiced in a high volume two stage custom juicer. First the grass blades are pulverized, then a press squeezes out all the liquid (juice), and it's off to the freezer where a harsh minus fifty degrees Fahrenheit (-45°C.) freezes the juice in under thirty minutes. This locks in all the nutrients and enzymes. Then all the air is sucked out creating a vacuum and the temperature is warmed to a balmy negative twenty degrees (-29°C.). In this environment the water molecules from the grass ice are drawn to the much colder condensing coil through a process called sublimation. Since the juice is ninety-six percent water, when sublimation is complete, only the grass solids remain. One hundred pounds of grass juice condense down to four pounds of grass solids. This concentrate holds the enzymes and nutrients in suspension until they are reactivated by adding water.

The wafer-like concentrate is then reduced to flakes in a climate controlled clean-room and automatically added into HDPE (#2 on the bottom) plastic bottles. There are no additives, fillers, binders or preservatives— just 100 percent pure freeze dried, certified organic (and Kosher, too) wheatgrass juice concentrate. When you look at it, it sparkles in the light. Its tiny crystals remind you of snowflakes. They grind it to a smooth powder for filling capsules and each capsule bottle includes a desiccant to reduce moisture that could have entered during the encapsulation process. Believe it or not, even though it is the same grass, you won't find the word "organic" on the front of the capsule bottle, only in small print on the back. This is because the veggie caps, made from cellulose, make up a little more than twenty percent of the product weight. Even though that cellulose may be more preferable to you than the gelatin capsules derived from cattle bones and pigskins, it is not certified organic. Therefore, while the powder bottle loudly proclaims its "organic-ness" on the front, the capsules bottle quietly speaks it on the back. One is 100 percent organic; the other is only about eighty. The products are good for one year. You can extend their shelf life beyond that by storing it in the freezer. This is one company where all growing, juicing, and packaging are done under one roof. If you can't find the product in your local store, visit their website and have it shipped direct to you.

Kyo-Green

Wakunaga of America Co. Ltd. Mission Viejo, California

800-421-2998. 714-855-2776. Fax 714-458-2764. www.kyolic.com

Wakunaga is a Japanese–American company originally established in Japan in 1955 with its American division located in Mission Viejo, California since 1986. This company is best known for Kyolic, the famous odorless aged garlic extract. It has a small line of botanicals, demonstrating its commitment to a selected group of herbs and phytochemicals. Wakunaga is not a grower of grasses nor do they produce a 100 percent grass product but they are listed here because they are a longtime player in the grass foods world and have a substantial presence on the market. They also have a reputation for quality. In 1991, Mr. Wakunaga was honored with Japan's Minister of Science and Technology award.

Their Kyo-Green is a grass combination product described as the best of land and sea. Wheat and barley grasses are grown for Wakunaga in the pristine Nasu highlands of Japan. Both are harvested at the jointing stage and combined with a premium chlorella. Chlorella is a single cell algae, cultivated by man that is two to three percent chlorophyll—the richest source on the planet. (Grasses and alfalfa are a close second.)

Chlorella is fifty-five to sixty-five percent protein by weight, making this a superb protein powder. The product also includes northern Pacific grown kelp and brown rice. The rice serves as a carbohydrate and fiber necessary for the spray drying of the juice. Kyo-Green melts readily in water or juice and has a smooth taste. In addition to the full spectrum of nutrients found in grasses, this blend is an especially good source of vitamin B-12, protein and iodine.

NaturesGreenz - New Zealand

NatureSource Organics Ltd. 0800-400-900. 64-9-270 0359, fax 64-9-270 0291. Onehunga, Auckland. <u>www.NaturesGreenz.com</u>

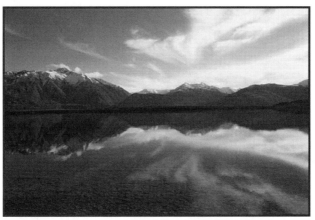

NaturesGreenz grown at the foot of the Southern
Alps in pristine South Island of New Zeland.

With all the air pollution, radiation, pesticides, and genetic engineering these days, it is hard to find a pristine growing environment. Traces of pesticides have even been found in certified organic foods. It's all because of the insidious spread of global pollution. But when it comes to wheatgrass, you need purity and quality because people depend on it for therapy. If there is any place on earth left in pristine condition, you could argue that it is in the South Pacific at the foot of the Southern Alps on the fertile Canterbury plains of New Zealand.

This is where *Nature's Greenz*™ grows its wheat and barley grasses on 500 unpolluted acres. At around forty-five degrees latitude, this is about as far south as you can go. The next stop is Antartica! It's a GE free zone here (no genetic modified grains), and radiation free as well. (New Zealand is a nuclear-free zone.) It's all certified by *IFOAM* the internationally recognized organic certifier and also by New Zealand's own certifier *AgriQuality*.

This relatively new company was founded by New Zealander Colin Middleton. Colin is an environmentalist, not a farmer. He started the company because of his research into cancer. He became convinced that the availability of high quality, affordable wheat and barley grasses could save lives.

Nature's Greenz blends both wheat and barley grasses together in all of its products. Their philosophy is that these two greens are similar and complementary. They see no need to differentiate and want their customers to benefit from both.

This is a whole leaf product, not a juice. During the growing season, crops are harvested every ten to twelve weeks. A mechanical harvester snips the young grass like a giant hedge trimmer at a height of approximately eight to nine inches (200mm). This is all done from November to May. That's their warm season. The rest of the year, the ground is covered with a foot of snow. The grass is then cleaned and milled into a fine powder. In fact, it is milled so finely, with a 0.6mm screen (0.002inch), that it mixes well in drinks and is easy to digest.

Organic crops universally have high microbial plate counts because no pesticides are used and organic companies would never consider such conventional treatments as irradiation and chlorine. So to protect the consumer from bacteria, including e-coli and salmonella, every batch is treated with a dry-steam purifier (the grass doesn't get wet) at fifty-five degrees Celsius (131°F.). It is purified for five minutes and then dehydrated in a tumble dryer at the same temperature for thirty minutes, thereby yielding a low moisture content of approximately four percent. Each batch is then sent to the laboratory for final testing. This meets organic standards and ensures the product is safe. Needless to say, this product uses no artificial colors, flavors, fillers, preservatives, sugar, milk, starch, gluten, or yeast derivatives. As a whole leaf food, it is also a superb source of vegetable fiber.

VitaRich Foods

Naples, Florida 800-817-9999, fax 941-591-8220 www.VitaRich.net

Vita-Rich started in 1992 and although fairly new on the scene, it has become a major player. This company is unique in that it does not produce its own brand. Instead it is the manufacturer behind the scenes of several popular grass and green food mixtures in the U.S., England, Australia and South Africa. Vita-Rich's main products are barley and wheatgrass, but it also cultivates a mineral-rich macro algae called Hydrillia.

Although headquartered in beautiful Naples Florida, its farm operation lies on the Northern Florida–Georgia border near Tallahassee. This provides a perfectly cool climate for wheat and barley. Their 2,500 acre farm has a high clay content that is ideal for mineral and moisture retention. Fertilizers stay on top longer, feeding the developing roots rather than percolating down beyond their reach. The fields are irrigated from an 800 foot deep well that delivers a rich mineral water. Three hundred acres of grain are planted and harvested from November through April. A laser sighting system helps level the land or angle it slightly for drainage. This smooth surface enables the harvester to get really close to the ground. The grass is cut just before jointing stage when the blades are about eight to nine inches tall. The young, sweet blades are soft and luscious and free of hard stalk fiber. When the stalk starts to develop, it creates a *seed head,* which drains the nutrients from the blades. This was the discovery of Charles Schnabel (see *The Pioneers*). Vita-Rich is able to get two cuttings per location before jointing.

Processing the Grass

Harvesters carefully convey the grass to the processing plant that is centrally located on the acreage. There the grass is put through a five tank washing system that includes ozonation to control microbe activity. Then the grass is dried and ground.

Their low-temperature 89°F drying system consists of a six foot wide conveyer that rides the grass leaves through a high volume dehumidifier over and over again until all the water is evaporated. It can take four hours or more to dry. This is longer than any other manufacturer because Vita-Rich president, Kevin Thomas, insists on drying the whole, intact leaf. "The more we crush, pulverize, or even bruise the leaves, the more we lose enzymatic activity. Drying the leaf whole keeps it fresher. It even smells better this way."

Once the leaf is dry and brittle, it can be powdered with less risk to its nutrition. Vita-Rich sucks the grass through a milling head that is kept to a cool 50°F with nitrogen. This protects against the higher temperatures generated by friction. The grass blades bounce and spin around until they become small enough to travel through the filter. By this time it has become a micro-fine particle that easily dissolves.

No Juice But You Won't Notice

Vita-Rich used to make grass juice using a spray dryer system like that developed by Hagiwara. But Thomas did not like all the mastication and pulverization of the plant along with the starch additives necessary as a carrier. He found that just grinding up the whole leaf was simpler, healthier and less expensive for the consumer. The Vita-Rich grinding method creates such fine particles, they dissolve nearly the same as a juice powder. Since grass is mostly water anyway, getting the few solids out creates more processing, more expense and more risk to the nutritional integrity of the plant than it's worth. Other companies cited in this chapter also take this approach.

> *This is a juice and fiber concentrate. It has 100% of juices and solid fiber minerals, enzymes, and proteins that are attached to the plant fiber cells. It dissolves readily because it is micro-pulverized. And it hasn't been diluted by the additives necessary for making juice powders.* —Kevin Thomas, Vita-Rich

Since Vita-Rich does not produce its own brand, safe transportation to the various manufacturers is required. The dried grass powder is shipped by Styrofoam insulated air freight containers and arrives the next day even in places as far away as South Africa. By land, it travels in insulated, air-conditioned trucks.

Vita-Rich does one more thing that is very unique. It uses strong magnets during the grinding stage to align the atoms of grass in a uniform polarity. Although this is an esoteric goal, it is based on immutable laws of physics. The concept is that properly polarized food will be handled more efficiently by the body, achieving more complete combustion and greater absorption. This is the same concept embraced by Tribest's GreenStar wheatgrass juicers (see *The Juicers*). Since grass customers are somewhat esoteric to begin with, this should not be a stretch for them. The magnets also have a practical application in that they eliminate static electricity built up from processing. Magnets are already popular in the health movement therapeutically for relief of pain, on home water systems for treatment of hard water, on auto fuel lines for improving gas mileage and in acupuncture treatment.

Greens Plus®

Orange Peel Enterprises. Vero Beach, Florida

800-643-1210, fax 561-562-9848. www.greensplus.com

Greens+® is the original grass and superfoods combination product. Looking at the dozens of green super-food powders on the market today, it is hard to believe that in 1992 there weren't any. But that is the year that Sam Graci premiered Greens+. Graci, author of *The Power of Superfoods*, is a chemist and psychologist by profession. In the 1970s, he worked with a group of Down Syndrome teens attempting to improve their social interactive skills. In the process, he discovered they had extreme vitamin, mineral, and enzyme deficiencies. Upon improving their diet and adding rest and exercise, he saw dramatic changes. Graci continued to do nutritional research with help from some very important experts including Dr. Linus Pauling. He wanted something that would be easier for people to take, rather than dozens of bottles of different colored vitamins. The result was an easy-to-mix powdered blend of super-foods. Graci believed that a concentrated whole food with its full spectrum of nutritional cofactors was more effective than isolated vitamins. The result was a synergistic blend of enzymatically active, alkaline-forming, nutrient-rich foods in an easy-to-take powder. At its foundation are barley and wheat grasses, along with alfalfa and the algaes—spirulina, chlorella, dulse and dunaliella. On top of this, he added organically grown soy sprouts, antioxidant herbs and extracts, probiotic cultures and pectins, royal jelly, ginseng and all in all, about twenty-nine different herbs and super-foods. He called this rich chlorophyll mixture Greens+ and arranged for Orange Peel Enterprises to manufacture it. Today, every major nutritional supplement manufacturer has its own version. Graci pioneered a new niche in the nutritional foods industry and barley and wheat grasses are the primary ingredients in every one of these products.

Although they now have much competition, Greens+ is still an industry leader. In 1996, they received the International Hall of Fame New Product award in the health category and took first place in the annual People's Choice Awards bestowed by the National Nutritional Foods Association. According to the Boston Herald, even David Letterman uses Greens+ and swears by it. These premium green foods raise energy levels, build mental acuity, strengthen the immune system, maintain colon ecology, balance pH, and enhance metabolism.

Perfect Foods, Inc.

4 Hawks Nest Road, Monroe, NY 10950

800-933-3288. www.800wheatgrass.com

There is an old saying about New York. If you can make it there you can make it anywhere. And it's true. New York wheatgrass users know their grass. They are savvy and fussy. Before they buy it, they examine the roots for mold, check for uniform green-ness; and make sure it is not too young or too old, nor too sweet or too tough. This is the environment under which *Perfect Foods* developed, and today it remains the oldest and largest wheatgrass grower in the New York City region. So when you see their fresh grass or their box of frozen wheatgrass juice in the freezer of your local health food store, you know it has passed the ultimate test. Although not in nationwide distribution, they are listed here because they are representative of the hundreds of regional wheatgrass growers who grow indoors and sell fresh grass to health food stores and consumers in their area. (For more regional growers, see *Resources.*)

Unlike outdoor growers who harvest only at select times, this grass is grown in small parcels and harvested every day of the year. But that's not all. The controlled indoor environment creates perfect light and temperature conditions for every crop, every day. This is peak performance gardening and it makes grass that is softer, longer, greener, juicier and sweeter. Experienced growers know that too much sun will make the grass tough and the juice foamy and less sweet. Walking into this growing room with its high intensity full-spectrum lights feels like a springtime afternoon on a partly cloudy day—just what the grass likes. Each parcel is inspected and juiced upon reaching its prime. Their juicer is a custom designed two step masticator that reduces oxidation to a minimum and presses the grass dry. Although the grass is grown in a controlled assembly line process, every parcel passes the human test from selection to tasting, to juicing and freezing. Workers pour the juice by hand into every one-ounce container–usually filling it higher than the one ounce mark–and freeze it rapidly in a huge, uniformly cold, blast freezer. From harvest to green ice, it is a fast couple of hours.

How does frozen grass compare to the fresh? No, the Journal of the American Medical Association did not perform a study. But grass users did. (See *Real Stories from Real People*.) Users growing in volume are often obliged to freeze their excess rather than let it grow past its prime. Those who are fighting illness depend on getting real results and their general consensus is that frozen is 90 percent as potent as fresh.

Evergreen Juices Inc.

P.O. Box # 1, Don Mills, Ontario, Canada M3C 2R6

905-709-2770, fax 905-709-2770. www.Evergreenjuices.com

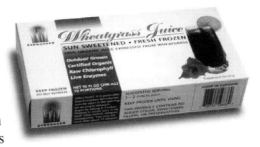

This "sun-sweetened" frozen grass juice is currently the only frozen grass juice sold in health stores in North America. All other field grass producers manufacture powdered grass products. Indoor grass growers, with few exceptions, provide fresh grass for juicing at juice bars or at home. Indoor and outdoor grasses have been compared elsewhere in this book *(see p. 92)*, but there is an irresistible temptation to combine the best of both worlds—the fresh living juice from indoor grass with the maturity, sunlight and deep soil of outdoor grass. Here is where *Evergreen*, stewarded by an eighty-four year young farmer, has taken the bold, creative initiative to fill that niche. True, you can't juice their grass in your home or get it at your juice bar, but as we've seen above, the frozen juice successfully suspends the living nutrients and comes pretty close to the fresh.

Evergreen plants its winter wheat and barley in southwestern Ontario in the fall and lets it grow for 200 days. The long winter allows the roots to suck up precious soil minerals. Once the spring sunshine and warmth arrive, those stored nutrients are transformed from simple sugars into complex carbohydrates, vitamins and proteins. The plants are harvested just before jointing stage *(see p. 43)* and the juice is extracted, chilled rapidly, and then frozen. Evergreen maintains that barley and wheat grass juices are virtually identical nutritionally when grown under the same conditions. Just defrost it; then sit back and drink in the liquid sunshine.

The Synergy Company™

800-723-0277, 435-259-5366, fax 435-259-2328

Moab, Utah   www.synergy-co.com

If you've ever had the pleasure of visiting Arches National Park, you know how incredibly unique this red dirt country is. Just outside the park is a wonderful sanctuary of progressive thinking and healthy living—the town of Moab, Utah. It is a fitting home for this company whose principles of quality and ethics match its pristine surroundings. Synergy is best known for *Pure Synergy®* its flagship superfood product. In it are wheat, barley, oat, and alfalfa grasses along with algaes such as spirulina, chlorella, Klamath blue-green, kelp, and others. It's about as green a drink as you'll get, and there are vegetables, wild crafted herbs, sprouts, and mushrooms included, as well. It is a connoisseur's blend of about sixty ingredients, but that is only part of the story. How these foods are grown and processed, from field to bottle, is a stunning example of diligence, technology, and devotion to nutrient preservation with a spare-no-expense attitude.

Freeze Drying

What sets this company apart from most of the others is its use of freeze drying technology. These machines, which cost about half a million dollars each, are the gold standard of drying equipment. Freeze drying occurs at below freezing temperatures in an oxygen-free (vacuum) environment. If you think about it, most drying equipment involves heat and air—two elements that are antagonistic to nutrients such as enzymes, antioxidants, carotenoids, and chlorophyll. Freeze-drying removes the water from the wheatgrass ice, without the ice ever melting. This process is called sublimation and it means the wheatgrass transforms from juice into crystals (solids) without warming and while remaining in

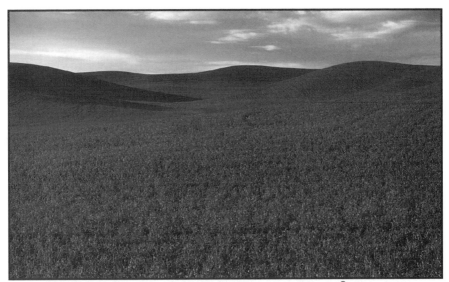

The Synergy Company's beautiful field of Synergized® wheatgrass
delivers active enzymes to you through its meticulous processing

a zero-oxygen environment. One thousand ounces of juice reduces to
only fifty ounces of freeze-dried wheatgrass crystals. There is only two
percent moisture left in the remaining solids, which is the maximum dehydration possible—any less and the product would become ash. It's not
only the quality of this method for nutrient preservation that is a benefit
here, but also the quantity of moisture. Since products are sold by weight,
if you think about it, when you buy a product with seven percent moisture, you are in part spending money on water. Synergy's 20:1 juice to
crystals ratio says it all. They deliver the wheatgrass essence. When you
get it home you can reconstitute it and add all the water or juice you want.

Actually, the quality considerations start long before the freeze-
dryer. Every step of the way marks an opportunity for degradation or
preservation. The grasses are grown in Northern California and the moment they are harvested, they are rushed by refrigerated truck to the processing plant where they are washed in cold water with a high oxygen
content. The oxygen doesn't hurt the blades; instead it kills bacteria and
purifies the grass. The grass is then sent to the juicer where a slow turning
spiral auger presses the juice from the blades. The juice is captured in
34°F. stainless steel tanks from which it is pumped into a blast freezer
that turns it into solid ice within thirty minutes.

The ice transforms to solids in the freeze dryer and the crystal solids are then vacuum packed in special oxygen barrier bags for the refrigerated trip to the state of the art bottling facility in Moab, Utah. Inside this 100 percent wind powered facility is where the product is packaged in dark amber glass bottles. Why not plastic? Because oxygen molecules are actually small enough to penetrate many plastics. So even though plastic bottles cost less than glass and are less expensive to ship, the choice was made in favor of nutrient preservation over cost. Inside each bottle is an oxygen absorbent and moisture absorbent (desiccant). The bottle is hermetically sealed with a foil cover that is actually bonded to the glass so as to ensure that no oxygen or moisture can enter.

The finished product is certified organic and certified Kosher. The product is tested for microbes, nutrients, and enzymes. Microbes are a problem for organic juice powders because the powder is a fertile nutrient base for bacteria. But with the low moisture content, the avoidance of manure fertilizer, and the washing and cold temperatures at every stage, the bugs never have a chance.

At the same time that this exacting process keeps out the bugs, it keeps in the enzymes. Super-oxide Dismutase (SOD) is one of the most vulnerable enzymes so it is tested as a marker. If SOD survives, then so do the other enzymes. A high chlorophyll content is another good marker, because this oil-soluble nutrient is very susceptible to heat. If the chlorophyll is high, so are the other heat liable nutrients. Speaking of chlorophyll, Synergy has developed another dehydration process that is achieving record breaking chlorophyll levels. It is air drying in an atmosphere of carbon dioxide—no oxygen. This innovative process is another example of how the folks at Synergy are forever seeking higher ground. Stay tuned.

I have had some really wonderful guides in my life and I feel a tremendous amount of responsibility and accountability to be true to what I was given. There is no reason to give people supplements that don't help them. It's a rip off. There is no amount of money to make me do what I'm doing. I have to answer to a higher cosmic power than just money.

—Mitchel May

Science & Wheatgrass
The Quest for Confirmation

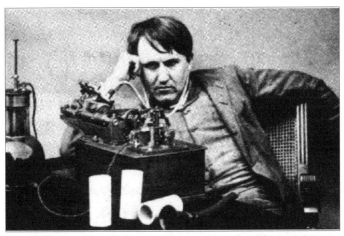

Thomas Alva Edison, after working for 60 straight hours perfecting the phonograph. As the inventor of the phonograph, motion picture, electric light and telephone enhancements, this man laid the foundation for the twentieth century.

Until Man duplicates a blade of grass, nature can laugh at his so called scientific knowledge. —Thomas Alva Edison

What role does science play in confirming wheatgrass as a natural medicine? In this book there are numerous research citations demonstrating its wondrous healing properties. Every decade since the 1930's has produced studies on its prodigious nutritional and phytochemical qualities. The magical properties of chlorophyll as a blood builder for the anemic, for disinfecting and neutralizing odors, and healing wounds started becoming known as far back as 1915. The 1970's, 80's and 90's presented numerous studies on barley grass and its superior antioxidant, tumor suppressant and immune supportive functions. These were traditionally designed studies with many published in peer-reviewed journals. Nevertheless, grasses are not a mainstream accepted food or medicine and their therapeutic potential benefits only a closed club of faithfuls. It is considered unproven. But clinical evidence from health professionals and testimony from users who have conquered life threatening diseases after being abandoned by conventional medicine have value. Do we need to wait until the therapeutic benefits of grass are scientifically proven before we use it?

Gray are all the theories, but Green is the Tree of Life. —Goethe

What Do You Believe?

Is all that is true only so because science has pronounced it? How are we to evaluate the "truth" without science? The extent of information we are willing to accept without scientific proof depends on our belief system.

Divine Belief. If you have a divine or intuitive belief system, then you trust in God and nature. You are likely to ask: "Do we have to understand why everything works before we try it?" *Faith* underlies the foundation of this belief system."And the truth shall bear witness of itself." "To feel beauty is a better thing than to understand how we come to feel it."—Santayana

Agnostic–Darwinian System. If you have an agnostic–Darwinian belief system, you require proof. You depend on science and are skeptical of anything unproven. "There is something Pagan in me that I cannot shake off. In short, I deny nothing, but doubt everything." —says Lord Byron, English poet (1811). "No scientist, however specialized his field, can factually accept even the Book of Genesis."—says Robert Graves, British novelist (1963).

What greater means of substantiation is better than scientific proof? Society does need a standard to measure things against. But science is a big world. Scientists themselves are frequently the first to look askance at the studies of other scientists. As a group, they are the ultimate skeptics. Even when proper protocol is followed, many still proclaim disbelief. If doctors and scientists dispute the results of studies, what are we as consumers supposed to believe? Throughout medical history, studies have contradicted one another and previously accepted positions have been reversed. In two recent studies on calcium, the title of the first read: *Calcium Supplementation Ineffective in Replacing Bone.* The second study, performed by a different group of scientists, but using the same protocol: the same diet, same number of people, same distribution of men and women, same ages, pronounced: *Calcium Effective in Replacing Bone.* Which one are we supposed to believe? It turns out that the only aspect of the two studies that was not identical was the source of the calcium. The first group used calcium carbonate, the second used calcium citrate.

The first group insisted: "calcium is calcium." But calcium carbonate is not readily absorbed by the body.

> *If the doctors and scientists don't agree, what are*
> *we consumers supposed to believe?*

Scientists still are not in agreement over the greenhouse effect. Yet according to the British Meteorological Service, 1995 was the warmest year in history. A United Nations panel of scientists predicts that if emissions are not reduced, climatic changes will become more and more irreversible. Are we to abide by the axiom: "If you can't prove it, it's not happening?" How sure do we have to be before changing the way we live? Dr. Charles F. Schnabel, a chemist to whom this book is dedicated, said upon discovering the phenomenal fertility of chickens eating wheatgrass: "I shall never forget the day in July, 1930 when I gathered 126 eggs from 106 hens. My first thought was— 'How long will it be before science can explain it?'"[3]

> *The art of healing comes from nature, not the physician.*
> *Therefore the physician must start from nature with an*
> *open mind.* —Paracelsus 1493–1541

Where Does Medicine Come From, Anyway?

It wasn't until the modern drug industry arose in the 19th century that medicines came from the laboratory. Nature is the original source of modern medicine. Pharmacopoeias of ancient Egypt, Babylonia, Greece, and China were based on food. Hippocrates, the father of modern medicine, proclaimed: "Let your food be your medicine and let your medicine be your food." The 12th century Jewish physician/philosopher Maimonides recommended chicken soup as a remedy for asthma. Garlic, mustard seed, and other herbs and spices were used medicinally for centuries. And what child doesn't know— "an apple a day keeps the doctor away." Many modern pharmaceuticals are actually synthetic replications of botanical products. Quinine from the cinchona tree was the only remedy for malaria for over 300 years. Penicillin, our first antibiotic, comes from mold. Aspirin is synthetic salicylic acid derived from the bark of the willow tree. In spite of our high technology, researchers today still look to nature for ideas and synthesize natural compounds. If nature is the source of all these miraculous medicines, why has it not earned our confidence? Why, as a society, can't we accept wheatgrass with the current level of proof? Even scientists believe in things. Indeed, they thrive on hunches. The only difference is that they substantiate their beliefs in the lab while we embrace them with our "faith."

> *Science without religion is lame. Religion without science is blind.* —Albert Einstein, 1934

> *The ordinary doctor is interested mostly in the study of disease. The nature doctor is interested mostly in the study of health.* —Mahatma Gandhi, 1869–1948.

Why Your Doctor Won't Tell You About Wheatgrass

We don't do very well with our differences in America. If one thing is good, the other has got to be bad. As a profession, medical doctors are automatic doubters. They cannot give wheatgrass credit, for to accept the existence of a significant medical force outside of their domain is to diminish their power. Every group has a natural instinct to protect itself. Is the doctors' position on wheatgrass an evaluation or a reaction? They must take an extreme position in the national arena. Their rhetoric is all black and white: Alternative medicine is filled with quacks and established medicine is the only valid system. The psychology is understandable but by taking this position, conventional medicine is protecting itself rather than protecting the public. What is this if not an intolerance for a different opinion? There are Nazi hate groups today that deny the occurrence of the holocaust. Does that mean it never happened? Is wheatgrass a fraud because the medical profession does not recognize it?

> *It is time we prove to America we are a doctors' organization, working for the good of our patients, rather than a pressure group aiming for political power as a way to build organizational predominance, to create personal prestige, or to line our own pockets.*
> —former AMA President, John J. Ring, MD.

Why There Aren't More Studies on Wheatgrass

Wheatgrass is not a drug. Natural products are not easily patented and the average cost of bringing a new product up to FDA approval is $359 million per therapeutic use. While this may be only a few days' earnings in the prescription drug industry, it is beyond the reach of natural products manufacturers. Getting a study published in medical journals is difficult, and drug companies have substantial political and financial influence with them, since journals depend on drug ads to survive. Unless the system changes, it is unlikely that approved medicines will come from anyone other than major pharmaceutical companies.

> *Any cure for cancer or anything else from outside the system must be suppressed to maintain the status quo.*

Conventional medicine takes years to accept any discovery that challenges cherished beliefs. Typically, a discovery that contradicts mainstream authority is regarded as quackery. Pasteur was reviled for years about his "germ theory." William Harvey (1628) was ridiculed when he claimed that blood circulates. Roentgen was laughed at in 1895 upon discovering X-rays. It is always an uphill fight opposing the status-quo which is, by its nature, against change.

> *Animals haven't heard anything about vitamins. They determine the nutritive value with their instinct, palate and olfactory faculties acting for them in place of judgement. The preferences shown by cattle are therefore better proofs than those obtained from the analysis of the chemist.*
> —George Sinclair, 1869

Approved Drugs Are Not So Safe

What critics often ignore is that not everything in conventional medicine is sanctioned by published science. Aspirin and penicillin became widely used long before experts knew how they worked. Many mainstream techniques such as surgery, anaesthesia and drugs are acknowledged as unsafe. In the April 1998 issue of the prestigious *Journal of the American Medical Association*, researchers calculated that adverse drug reactions may kill more than 100,000 Americans each year. In 1994, deaths from drug reactions were so numerous that statistically they placed between the fourth and sixth leading cause of death in the United States. What value are published studies and expensive FDA approval if this is the result? The FDA claims the "benefits of drugs outweigh the risks." Since wheatgrass has no known toxic side effects, it has no risks, just benefits. Yet, in spite of the rather deadly track record of approved drugs, wheatgrass is still rejected as untested and unproven.

Not All Studies are Valid

Every year FDA approved drugs are pulled off the market because of incidents involving dangerous side effects, including deaths. How valuable then, is government approval? How reliable are scientific studies if, as in the case of the two calcium studies, we cannot depend on the results? Can you interpret a scientific study? Since for most of us the answer to this is "no," then why do we place so much value in them? To protect ourselves, we must ask some questions.

How To Study A Study

What are the credentials of the scientists? Is it a double blind study where neither the patient nor the scientist know the source of the sample? Are placebos used? Has the study been published in a peer reviewed journal? Are the results statistically significant? Were the tests done in vivo or in vitro—in animals or in test tubes? On mice or people? Who funded it? Is there any group who will benefit from this financially? Are testimonials by doctors paid for? Look for a conflict of interest such as the cigarette industry financing a study on lung cancer. Beware of health claims that tout one product as a panacea. Health is never that simple.

Healing is Electrical, Spiritual, Chemical, Physical

Americans love pills. Modern medicine has provided us with some powerful effects through chemistry. The scientists and pharmacologists should be applauded for the powerful medicines they have developed. But healing is more than chemistry. Taking vitamins all day will not alone solve most chronic conditions. The restoration of health is complex. There is no magic pill. Wheatgrass is neither a pill nor a panacea. But when used as part of a total health revitalization program with an indefatigable commitment to wellness, it is a powerful healing agent that will maximize and accelerate your health potential.

Health is more than nutrition—more than the physical feeding of chemicals to cells. We are more than just physical, mechanical bodies. We are bio-electrical, spiritual beings inside physical bodies. One of the secrets to the effectiveness of wheatgrass is that it nourishes us on these levels, too. As a high vibration living food, it raises our chi to a higher vibratory level. In the drug culture's vernacular, you get high. It's the difference between walking and jogging. Wheatgrass accelerates the electrical activity inside every cell. That doesn't happen with canned carrots, powdered potatoes, french fries or microwave pizza. Chocolate makes you feel good because it temporarily spikes your blood sugar. Coffee is a chemical stimulant. But grass enlivens you. It's like charging your biological battery. It's a natural high, boosting your own manufacture of adrenalin. It's how you feel when you're on top of the world. You can conquer any challenge, defeat any foe. This is the spiritual factor that is a necessary part of any successful battle with illness. The Chinese call it chi; the yogi's call it kundalini—the God–force, the life force. With it behind you, you can go far and you can go fast. You are the healer. Wheatgrass is the energizer.

The Final Analysis

Although many people have heard about wheatgrass, it remains largely unknown and undiscovered in the general population. When you mention "grass" to the masses, they think you mean marijuana. But for the thousands who are turned away each day by conventional medicine, wheatgrass is hope, not dope. In the world of alternative medicine, grass is king. Whether or not you believe in it, it has earned the right to be evaluated by more people—before they enter a desperate health crisis. This book provides the tools to help you design your own alternative health rejuvenation program.

Wheatgrass is hope, not dope

Do you need scientific verification? That is a question you must answer for yourself. But a successful health journey must include faith. If you were to guess whether wheatgrass could benefit your health, what would your answer be? Take charge of the direction of your personal health journey. It is an illusion to believe that doctors, hospitals, scientists or anyone else knows better than you. You already have the knowledge to make the right decision. Now you need only muster the courage.

Sproutman®

Let's change "Impossible" to "I'm Possible."
—Dr. Bernard Jensen

If I have the belief that I can do it, I shall surely acquire the capacity to do it even if I may not have it at the beginning.
—Mahatma Gandhi

Epilogue
by Dr. Ann Wigmore

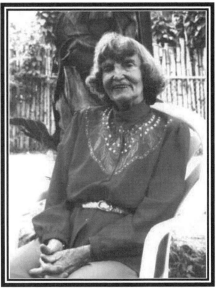

Ann Wigmore

Today in the twentieth century, we must learn to survive, not only from the hazards of pollution in our water and air, but also from our food supply itself. Many Americans are slowly killing themselves by what they eat each day. Thousands of chemical additives have found their way into our daily foods and the foods themselves are overcooked and overre-fined during processing, storage, delivery and marketing. Staples like bread and cereals are so depleted of their own naturally occurring vita-mins, minerals and bran by over-processing and refining, that laws have been passed forcing manufacturers to fortify them with synthetic ones.

Malnutrition amongst the world's affluent peoples is becoming more and more common. It is the natural result of eating too many foods which have been processed and cooked to the extent that they are depleted of their naturally occurring nutrients. However, we have a choice of how we want to live and what we want to put into our bodies.

For almost thirty years I have been teaching people all over the world how to grow their own highly nutritious live foods like sprouts, indoor garden greens and wheatgrass at less than half the cost of supermarket foods. I have also lived almost entirely on these foods which I grow from seed in my home in Boston and even while I am traveling.

It is easy to control your own food supply and take responsibility for one's health. Time has shown that our battles against degenerative and chronic diseases like cancer, heart disease, diabetes, arthritis and many others cannot be won by palliative measures like surgery, chemotherapy and other medical intervention, but only through prevention. Unfortunately, more people wait until there is a critical problem to give preventative action a thought and then it becomes a question of preventing a recurrence. But true prevention stops a problem before there is any serious permanent damage. The fact is survival is not only possible but joyous. It is the re-inheritance of our natural birthright–health–which has been stripped from us by modern man's errors in judgement.

—*Ann Wigmore*, Boston, 1984.

Ann Wigmore died in Boston on February 16, 1994, in the Mansion where she taught, of smoke inhalation from an electrical fire. She was 84.

The Ann Wigmore Foundation is now located at PO Box 399, San Fidel, NM 87049. 505-552-0595. Her retreat center in Puerto Rico is the Ann Wigmore Institute, PO Box 429, Rincon, PR 00743, 787-868-6307.

References and Studies

HISTORY AND CULTURE

1. Biogenic Meditation Biogenic Self-Analysis Creative Micro-Cosmos. Students' and Teachers' Digest and Guidebook to Intensive Biogenic Seminars. International Biogenic Society. 1978. See Resources: I.B.S. and Awareness Institute.

2. *Grasses An Identification Guide*, by Lauren Brown. Houghton Mifflin, 1979.

3. Ibid

4. *Hortus Gramineus Woburnensis* or, an Account of the Results of Experiments on the Produce and Nutritive Qualities of Different Grasses, used as the Food of the More Valuable Domestic Animals. By George Sinclair, Gardener to the late Duke of Bedford. Instituted by John Duke of Bedford. Published by Ridgways. London, 1869. 362 pages.

5. Kellner, Jordan, Wilson, et al. Missouri, 1915. From The Cause and Cure of Famine and Hidden Hunger, by Charles F. Schnabel. 1936. Unpublished.

6. Second Annual Report of the Department of Agriculture state of New Hampshire, 1890 by Morse, F.W.

7. Woodman, H.E. & associates. *Journal of Agricultural Science*, 1925–1930.

8. *Hortus Gramineus Woburnensis*. (See previous note) By George Sinclair. London, 1869.

SPIRITUAL AND RELIGIOUS ROOTS

1. Song of Myself by Walt Whitman, 1819-1892, sct. 31, in *Leaves of Grass* (1855).

2. *George Washington Carver–An American Biography* by Rackham Holt. Doubleday, Doran & Co., 1943.

3. *The Meaning of the Word Grass in Hebrew*. Published by The Western Wheatgrass Journal, VII, No. 1. Jan-Mar. 1995. 3353 South Main, Salt Lake City, UT 84115. *See Resources.*

4. *Written By the Finger of God—Decoding Ancient Languages*, by Joe Sampson, Oct. 1993. Wellspring publishing, Box 1113 Sandy UT 4091. ISBN 1884312-05-5.

5. Op.cit.

6. See chapter: *Nutrition*

7. Conversation with Piter U. Caizer, by Steve Meyerowitz, California, March 15, 1998. Edited by Steve Meyerowitz. All rights reserved. Permission for use in any medium is required.

8. Ibid.

9. *The Essene Gospel of Peace Book IV*, by Edmond Bordeaux Szekely. Chapter: "The Gift of the Humble Grass." International Biogenic Society. Used with permission.

10. *International Biogenic Society.* P.O. Box 849, Nelson, B.C. Canada V1L 6A5. www.thenazareneway.com

11. *The Essene Gospel of Peace Book IV*, by Edmond Bordeaux Szekely. Chapter: "The Gift of the Humble Grass." International Biogenic Society. Used with permission.

12. Extracted from "*Grass is the Forgiveness of Nature.*" The author was the senator from Kansas in the late 1890's.

THE PIONEERS

1. *Letter to Conrad A. Elvehjem*, July 10, 1942. Personal papers.

2. "*The Place of 40% Protein Grass in Modern Agriculture*," by C.F. Schnabel. Unpublished papers. 1939.

3. "*Good Grass is the Basis of A Permanent Agriculture*," by C.F. Schnabel.

4. "*Peace from Grass*" by C.F. Schnabel, B.S., D.Sc. Cappers Farmer, October, 1947.

5. JAMA. *Journal of the American Medial Association.* "Council on Foods: Accepted Foods." Franklin C. Bing, Secretary 1939. 112:733.

6. *The Relation of the Grass Juice Factor to Guinea Pig Nutrition.* By G.O. Kohler, C.A. Elvehjem, and E.B. Hart, Department of Agriculture Chemistry, University of Wisconsin, Madison. Journal of Nutrition, Vol.15, No.5. 11/24/1937

7. "The Amazing Anti-Aging Diet," by Claudia D. Bowe, *Cosmopolitan*, November, 1983.

8. *The Hippocrates Diet and Health Program*, by Ann Wigmore. Avery Publishing Group, Wayne, NJ. 1984. Dennis Weaver, actor from forward, regarding Dr. Ann's book.

9. *How I conquered Cancer Naturally*, by Eydie Mae Hunsberger and Chris Loeffler. Harvest House Publishers.

10. *The Wheatgrass Book*, by Ann Wigmore. Avery Publishing Group.

11. *Young Barley Plant Juice*, by Yoshihide Hagiwara, M.D. pub. by The Green and Health Association, Tokyo, Japan April, 1980.

12. *Ann Wigmore Foundation.* PO Box 399, San Fidel, NM 87049. 505-552-0595.

13. *Green Barley Essence: The Ideal Fast Food*, by Yoshihide Hagiwara, New Canaan, CT. Keats Publishing, Inc. 1986.

14. *Young Barley Plant Juice*, by Yoshihide Hagiwara, M.D. pub. by The Green and Health Association, Tokyo, Japan April, 1980.

NUTRITION

1. Dr. Charles F. Schnabel, father of wheatgrass in a letter to scientist Conrad A. Elvehjem, discoverer of niacin, July 10, 1942.

2. *The Cause and Cure of Famine and Hidden Hunger.* 1936. Charles F. Schnabel. Unpublished.

3. Phillips & Goss. Journal Agricultural Research. Vol. 51:p. 301. 1935.

4. *Chlorophyll. Nature's Green Magic* by Theodore M. Rudolph, Ph.D. Nutritional Research Publishing Company. PO Box 489, San Gabriel, CA. 1957.

5. Food Science for All, New Sunlight Theory of Nutrition. E. Bircher, Health Research Press.

6. Chlorophyll and Hemoglobin Regeneration After Hemmorrhage, by J.H. Hughes and A.L. Latner. Journal of Physiology. Vol.86, #388, 1936 University of Liverpool.

7. Chlorophyll, Nature's Green Magic, Dr. Theodore Rudolph.

8. The Influence of Diet on the Biological Effects Produced by Whole Body Irradiation. M. Lourou, O. Lartigue, Experientai, 6:25, 1950.

9. Further Studies on Reduction of X-irradiation of Guinea Pigs by Plant Materials. Quartermaster Food and Container Institute for the Armed Forces Report. N.R. 12-61. by D.H. Colloway, W.K. Calhoun, & A.H. Munson. 1961.

HEALING WITH GRASS

1. The Wheatgrass Book by Dr. Ann Wigmore, Avery Publishing Group, Garden City Park, NY.

2. Performed at Hippocrates Health Institute in the 1970's by Ann Wigmore and staff.

3. See: *Juice Fasting and Detoxification* by Steve Meyerowitz. 1996. ISBN#1-878736-65-5.

4. The Place of 40% Protein Grass in Modern Agriculture, by C.F. Schnabel. Unpublished. 1939.

5. Numerous cookbooks are available for juice recipes including "Sproutman's Kitchen Garden Cookbook," and "Power Juices Super Drinks" by this author. ISBN# 1-878736-86-8 and ISBN# 1-57566-528-X. See "Other Books" at the rear of this book.

6. Journal of Personality and Social Psychology, June 1998. By S.C. Segerstrom, University of Kentucky in Lexington, Psychology dept.

7. Science Newsletter, 1941 by Dr. R. Redpath and T.C. Davis.

8. Chlorophyll: An Experimental Study of its Water-Soluble Derivatives in Wound Healing. by L.W. Smith and A.E. Livingston. American Journal of Surgery. 52:358, 1943.

REAL STORIES FROM REAL PEOPLE

1. Courtesy of *The Wheatgrass & Sprouting Journal*. 3353 South Main, Suite 197, Salt Lake City, UT 84115.

2. Mr. Lampro was a student at *Hippocrates Health Institute* in West Palm Beach, Florida (*see Retreats*) where he established his wheatgrass and health program.

3. Russell Rosen, director of the former Naples Institute of Optimum Health & Healing.

4. Julian Whitaker, MD is editor of the *Health and Healing Newsletter*, the largest natural health newsletter in the world. He is also author of *New Cures for Chronic Diseases*, which is available free to newsletter subscribers. He operates the *Whitaker Wellness Institute* in Newport Beach, CA. To receive the *Health and Healing Newsletter* call 800-539-8219. To find out more about the *Whitaker Wellness Institute*, call 800-826-1550.

5. The Place of 40% Protein Grass in Modern Agriculture by C.F. Schnabel, Ph.D. Unpublished papers. 1939.

6. Philippus Paracelsus, 1493–1541, was a German born physician who introduced the concept of disease to medicine.

WHEATGRASS RETREATS

1. The Hippocrates Diet and Health Program by Ann Wigmore. Avery Publishing Group, 1984.

THE COMPANIES

1. Even the space taken to discuss these companies should not be construed as an indirect recommendation. It is more likely related to the history and longevity of the company and the depth of the materials available about them.

2. Consumer testimonial courtesy of Pines International, Inc.

3. Kamut is a registered trademark of Kamut International Ltd. of Fort Benton, Montana and is listed with the Department of Agriculture as QK77. www.kamut.com

Resources
Where to Go to Get Wheatgrass, Related Products, and Information

*For the latest information, visit
"Wheatgrass and Sprouts" at <u>www.Sproutman.com</u>*

Mail Order Grass Growers & Shippers

Sproutman.com. 413-528-5200, fax 413-528-5201. Wheatgrass products such as fresh organic grass and sprouts shipped nationwide; wheatgrass juice powders, extracts, creams, and sprays. Organic sprouting seeds. Automatic wheatgrass growers, sprouting bags, and related books. www.Sproutman.com

Gourmet Greens. 802-875-3820 ext. 4. 866-616-8698. Chester, Vermont. Next day delivery of certified organic wheatgrass and sprouts plus seeds and supplies to grow your own. Wheatgrass and vegetable juicers. Richard Rommer proprietor; grew grass for Ann Wigmore at the original *Hippocrates Health Institute*. www.Gourmetgreens.com

Wheatgrass Express. 800-859-4779, fax 386-462-7398. Gainesville, Florida. Certified organic grass delivered fresh overnight to your door. Also shipping "grow your own" wheatgrass kits. Wheatgrass grown with the mineral rich ocean fertilizer, Ocean Grown. www.wheat-grass.com

Perfect Foods. 800-933-3288, fax 845-651-2262. Monroe, NY. Oldest and largest fresh wheatgrass supplier in New York. Wheatgrass juicers and frozen grass juice. www.800wheatgrass.com

Monocot Wheatgrass. Toll-free 877-699-4328, 512-272-8700. Wheatgrass supplies, kits, troubleshooting help and instruction. Ships grass flats within Texas. www.austinwheatgrass.com

Dynamic Greens. 1-877-843-9452. 905-910-0467. Stouffville, Ontario. Canadian and U.S. grower-shipper of frozen outdoor grown wheatgrass juice. www.dynamicgreens.com

Sun Grown Organics Distributors, Inc. 800-995-7776. San Diego, California. One of California's largest and oldest growers and shippers of fresh wheatgrass and sprouts. www.sungrownorganics.com

Door to Door Organics. 888-283-4443. Pipersville, PA. Ships fresh wheatgrass and organic foods. www.doortodoororganics.com

Diamond Organics. 888-674-2642. Moss Landing, California. Ships fresh wheatgrass, organic foods, and sprouts. www.diamondorganics.com

WheatgrassExpress.com. 866-583-8776. Fresh wheat and barley grass, wheatgrass kits and juicers. www.wheatgrassexpress.com

International Resources

Bondi Wheatgrass Juice Company. 02-9694-1100, fax 02-9694-1177. One Dacre Street, Malabar, NSW, Australia 2036. Full service organic wheatgrass supplier. www.bondiwheatgrass.com.au

Sprout Organic Wheatgrass. Australia. Tel: 1300-79-30-70, Wheatgrass juicers, seeds and growing kits. Also sponsors of the educational site www.wheatgrasshealth.info www.sprout.net.au

Swheat! Wheatgrass shots. Live Liquids Pty Ltd, Sydney Australia. 61-1300-swheat, 61-417-658-090. Swheat! is an innovative wheatgrass company selling ready-to-drink wheatgrass shots. They have a shelf life of 12 days or more. www.Swheat.com.au

NatureSource Organics Ltd. New Zealand. 0800-400-900. 64-9-270 0359, fax: 64-9-270 0291. Onehunga, Auckland. Major grower and bottler of barley and wheatgrass. www.NaturesGreenz.com

Wheatgrass Pty. Ltd. Melbourne, Australia. +61-3-9827-6284. Fax+61-3-9827-6293. Manufacturer of a shelf stable wheatgrass drink, therapeutic extract, sprays, and creams. www.DrWheatgrass.com.au

Organically Grown Wheatgrass. Australia. Suppliers of fresh trays of Certified Organic Wheatgrass in Melbourne and Victoria. 0429-805-771.

Mumm's. Saskatchewan, Canada. 306-747-2935. Supplier of organic wheatgrass seed, and other sprouting seeds. www.sprouting.com

Healthmakers. Utrecht, SA +27 34 331 4824, Tel (SA) 0861 100 695. Wheatgrass growing kits and sprouters. www.healthmakers.co.za

Aquilahealth. South Africa. Wheatgrass juicers and sprouters. Tel: +2711 704-4949, Fax: +2711 704-6262. www.aquilahealth.co.za

InnerGarden Wheatgrass. Edmonton, Alberta. Canada. 780-432-3424. 888-299-3807. Fresh & frozen grass. www.innergardenwheatgrass.com

The UK Centre for Living Foods. +44(0)1584-875308. Wheatgrass and live foods classes in the UK. www.livingfoods.co.uk

Keimling Naturkost GmbH. Germany. +49(0)4161-5116-12, Fax +49(0)4161-5116-16. 21614 Buxtehude. Supplier of wheatgrass and barleygrass juice powders and juicers. www.keimling.de

Green Connection. Germany. 97516 Oberschwarzach. 09382-7879, fax 09382-7886. Fresh wheatgrass. www.weizengras.de

Savant. Leeds, UK. 44-113-388-5230. Distributors of wheatgrass and barleygrass juice powders and juicers. www.juicersonline.co.uk

Alpha Health Products of Canada. 800-663-2212. 604-436-0545. Brunaby, BC. Plastic freezer bags for freezing wheatgrass juice into cubes. Wheatgrass juicers and sprouters. www.alphahealth.ca

Growers and Manufacturers

Pines International, Inc. 800-MY-PINES (800-697-4637), Fax 785-841-1252. Lawrence, Kansas. www.wheatgrass.com

Green Foods Corporation. 800-777-4430, fax 805-983-8843. Oxnard, California. Green Magma and barley grass juice. www.greenfoods.com

Greens Plus. 800-643-1210, fax 561-562-9848. Orange Peel Enterprises, Inc. Vero Beach, Florida. www.greensplus.com

Evergreen Juices Inc. 905-886-8090, 1-877-91JUICE. Don Mills, Ontario, Canada. Major wheatgrass grower supplying frozen juice cubes at health stores in North America www.EvergreenJuices.com

Sheldon Farm, LLC. Chaplin, Conn. 866-974-3375 fax 860-974-2836. Greenhouse-grown, freeze-dried wheatgrass juice. www.SheldonFarm.com

Synergy Production Laboratories. Moab, Utah. 435-259-4787. Contract manufacturer of dried grass juice products. www.synergy-co.com

Sonne, V.E. Irons. 800-544-8147, 816-221-3719. Kansas City, MO. Makers of the GreenLife grass juice since 1953. www.veirons.com

Dynamic Nutraceuticals. 877-396-2473. PO Box 940, Sebastopol, CA 95473. Freeze-dried wheatgrass juice. www.dyna-green.com

Amazing Grass. San Francisco, California. 415-722-5710. Growers and processors of whole leaf wheatgrass. www.AmazingGrass.com

Kyo-Green. Wakunaga of America Co. 800-421-2998, 714-855-2776, Mission Viegjo, California. Makers of Kyo-Green. www.kyolic.com

Wheatgrass Training Centers

Ann Wigmore Institute - Puerto Rico. USA. Tel 787-868-6307, fax 787-868-2430. PO Box 429, Rincon, PR 00677. On the beach, live-in wheatgrass clinic and living foods center. www.AnnWigmore.org

Ann Wigmore Foundation. 505-552-0595. San Fidel, New Mexico. Live-in educational wheatgrass retreat center teaching the Living Foods Lifestyle®. www.wigmore.org

Optimum Health Institute - San Diego. 800-993-4325. 619-464-3346, fax 619-589-4098. Lemon Grove, California. World's largest residential wheatgrass training center. www.optimumhealth.org

Optimum Health Institute - Austin, Texas. 800-993-4325, 512-303-4817, fax 512-303-1239. Cedar Creek, TX. Texas branch of the California live-in wheatgrass training center. www.optimumhealth.com

Hippocrates Health Institute. 561-471-8876. Resv. 800-842-2125. West Palm Beach, Florida. World's most prestigious residential wheatgrass and raw foods training center. www.hippocratesinst.com

Hallelujah Acres. 800-651-7622, 704-481-1700. Shelby, North Carolina. Large Christian community focusing on raw vegetarian diet, including grasses and sprouts. Classes and events. Four residential Lifestyle Centers in FL, NC, TN, KY. www.halifestylecenters.com

Living Foods Institute. 800-844-9876, 404-524-4488. Atlanta, Georgia. Grass and live food classes. www.LivingFoodsInstitute.com

Creative Health Institute. 866-426-1213, 517-278-6260. Union City, Michigan. Residential living foods and wheatgrass training center following the Ann Wigmore program. www.creativehealthinstitute.com

Assembly of Yahweh Living Foods. 517-663-1637. Eaton Rapids, Michigan. A new Living Foods Lifestyle residential center with beds to accommodate five guests. www.assemblyofyahweh.com

Tree of Life Center. 866-394-2520. 520-394-2520. Patagonia, Arizona. Spiritual, eco-retreat center with organic Kosher live-food cuisine, sprouts and wheatgrass. Consultations with Dr. Gabriel Cousens, recognized medical doctor and author. www.treeoflife.nu

Seed Sources

Catalog for Healthy Eating. Summertown, Tenn. 800-695-2241. Wheatgrass and Sproutman's Organic Sprouting Seeds. Wheatgrass kits, automatic sprouters, liquid kelp, hydrogen peroxide, raw foods, sprout books and supplies. www.healthy-eating.com/sproutseeds.html

WheatgrassKits.com. Springville, Utah. 801-491-8700, Fax 801-491-8728. The original and largest wheatgrass kit manufacturer in the world. Full line of wheatgrass supplies. www.wheatgrasskits.com

The Sprout House. 800-777-6887. Wheatgrass and barley grass kits, EasyGreen sprouter, seeds and supplies. www.SproutHouse.com

Johnny's Selected Seeds. 207-437-4357, fax 800-437-4290. Albion, Maine. Organic gardening and sprouting seeds. www.Johnnyseeds.com

Optimum Health Institute. 800-993-4325. 619-464-3346. Sprouting Seeds and supplies. www.optimumhealth.org

Organic Provisions. 800-490-0044. Mail order supplier of organic and natural foods including some sprouting seeds. www.orgfood.com

Sproutpeople. 877-777-6887. San Francisco, California. Wheatgrass seeds and growing kits. www.sproutpeople.com

Grow Wheatgrass. 805-684-4071. Carpinteria, California. Multi-Shelf wheatgrass growing units. Soil or non-soil. www.growwheatgrass.com

General

Sproutman. The author gives private consultations on wheatgrass therapy, digestive problems, diet changes, juicing, fasting, and related topics. 413-528-5200, fax 413-528-5201. www.Sproutman.com

Michael Bergonzi. Master wheatgrass grower and consultant. Greenhouse director for Hippocrates Health Institute in Florida. wheatgrassking@yahoo.com www.hippocratesgreenhouse.com

Loreta's Living Foods. 610-648-0241. Consultations on living foods and wheatgrass therapy by an experienced teacher who worked with Dr. Ann Wigmore. www.loretaslivingfoods.com

Seed & Grain Technologies. 505-255-1555, fax 505-255-1554. Albuquerque, New Mexico. Manufacturers of Easy-Green, a hydroponic wheatgrass and sprout grower. www.easygreen.com

New Life Systems. 989-689-0005. Rhodes, Michigan. Do-it-yourself, homebuilt hydroponic wheatgrass sprouter kit and other raw foods tools. www.eatsprouts.com

Karyn's Fresh Corner. 3351 N. Lincoln Avenue, Chicago, IL 60657. 312-255-1590. Gourmet raw food restaurant and classes by this celebrated raw foods teacher. Wheatgrass juice bar. Treatment center with a variety of services on premises. www.karynraw.com

Rhio's Raw Energy Hotline. A raw/live foods help line and resource directory of classes and events in the New York metro area and beyond. Ask for Rhio's new raw foods cookbook. www.rawfoodinfo.com

San Francisco Living Foods Enthusiasts. 415-751-2806. San Francisco, CA. Telephone help line and listing of live foods pot-lucks, lectures and events in the San Francisco area. www.rawfoods.com/sflife

AgriGenic Food Corp. 800-788-1084, fax 714-899-0078. Huntington Beach, California. Manufacturer of live enzyme and antioxidant supplements from young wheat sprouts. www.agrigenic.com

OceanGrown. 941-921-2401. Sarasota, Florida. Liquid sea minerals for enriching your soil or soil-free garden. www.oceangrown.com

International Sprout Growers Association. 800-448-8006. Professional trade association for commercial sprout and grass growing. www.ISGA-Sprouts.org

Kamut Association of North America. Great Falls, Montana. 1-800-644-6450. 406-452-7227, fax 406-452-7175. www.kamut.com

Juicer Manufacturers

The Green Power Juicer. 888-254-7336. Los Angeles, California. Manufacturer of Tribest twin gear juicers. www.greenpower.com

Omega Juicers. 800-633-3401, fax 717-561-1298. PO Box 4523, Harrisburg, PA 17111. www.omegajuicers.com

L'Equip. 800-816-6811. 717-730-7100, fax 717-730-7200. 555 Bolser Ave., Harrisburg, PA 17043. www.lequip.com

Miracle Exclusives, Inc. 800-645-6360, fax 516-933-4760. 205 Park Ave, Hicksville, NY 11801. www.MiracleExclusives.com

Sundance Industries. Box 1446, Newburgh, New York 12550. 845- 565-6065, fax 845-562-5699 www.SundanceInd.com

Other Books about Grass

Cereal Grasses. by Ron Seibold. Pines International, Inc. 800-697-4637, fax 785-841-1252. PO Box 1107, Lawrence, KS 66044.

How I Conquered Cancer Naturally. by Eydie May Hunsberger. Penguin Publishing. ISBN 0-89529-518-0

The Wheatgrass Book. by Ann Wigmore. ISBN 0-89529-234-3

The Hippocrates Diet. by Ann Wigmore. ISBN 0-89529-223-8

Index

Other Books

By Steve Meyerowitz
www.Sproutman.com

The Organic Food Guide
How to Shop Smarter and Eat Healthier. 2004. $8.95

Water the Ultimate Cure
Discover Why Water is the Most Important Ingredient in your Diet and Find Out Which Water is Right for You. 2001. $7.95

Power Juices Super Drinks
Quick, Delicious Recipes to Reverse and Prevent Disease. 2000. $14

Sprouts the Miracle Food
The Complete Guide to Sprouting. 1999. $12.95

Food Combining and Digestion
101 Ways to Improve Digestion. 2002. $9.95

Sproutman's Kitchen Garden Cookbook
Sprout Breads, Cookies, Soups, Salads & 250 other Low Fat, Dairy Free Vegetarian Recipes. 1999. $14.95

Juice Fasting & Detoxification
Use the Healing Power of Fresh Juice to Feel Young and Look Great. 2002. $10.95

Sproutman's "Turn the Dial" Sprout Chart
A Field Guide to Growing and Eating Sprouts. 1998. $5.95

Clinician's Complete Reference to Complementary/ Alternative Medicine.
Steve Meyerowitz, co-author. Edited by Donald W. Novey, M.D. 2000.

Who Is This Sproutman®?

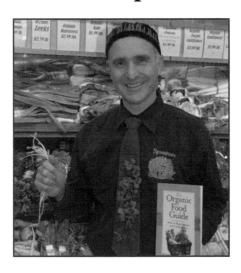

Steve Meyerowitz began his journey to better health in 1975 to correct a lifelong chronic condition of severe allergies and asthma. After almost twenty years of disappointment with conventional medicine, Steve restored his health through his own program of detoxification, yoga, fasting, juicing, exercise, lifestyle adjustment, and living foods. He became symptom-free in only two months.

Over the years, he has lived on and experimented with many so- called "extreme" diets, including: raw foods, fruitarianism, sprouts, dairyless and flourless vegetarianism, and liquitarianism. In 1977, he was pronounced "Sproutman" by *Vegetarian Times Magazine* in a feature article that explored his innovative sprouting ideas.

Steve opened *The Sprout House* a "no-cooking" school in New York City in 1980 where he shared his kitchen gardening techniques, cuisine, and recipes. He is the inventor of the fabric sprout bag, first made from flax and later hemp. A long-time health crusader, he has been featured on PBS, the Home Shopping Network, QVC, and the TV Food Network, as well as in magazines such as Organic Gardening, Prevention, House & Garden, and Better Nutrition.

Steve and his family, including three little sprouts, now live and breathe the fresh air in the Berkshire mountains of Massachusetts.